Legal Dangerous Drugs

The Poisons in your Medicine Chest

By **William Campbell Douglass**, M.D.

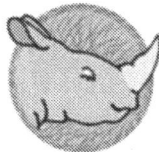

Rhino Publishing, S.A.

Legal Dangerous Drugs

The Poisons in your Medicine Chest

ISBN 9962-636-15-9

Cover illustration by
Alex Manyoma (alex@3dcity.com)

Please, visit Rhino's website for other publications from
Dr. William Campbell Douglass
www.rhinopublish.com

Dr. Douglass' "Real Health" alternative medical
newsletter is available at www.realhealthnews.com

RHINO PUBLISHING, S.A.
World Trade Center
Panama, Republic of Panama

Voicemail/Fax
International: + 416-352-5126
North America: 888-317-6767

Contents

Other Books by
William Campbell Douglass, MD

- *Add 10 Years To Your Life*
- *Aids And Biological Warfare*
- *Bad Medicine*
- *Color Me Healthy*
- *Dangerous Legal Drugs: The Poisons In Your Medicine Chest*
- *Dr. Douglass Complete Guide To Better Vision*
- *Eat Your Cholesterol! -- Meat, Milk, And Butter -- And Live Longer*
- *Grandma Bell's A To Z Guide To Healing*
- *Hormone Replacement Therapies: Astonishing Results For Men And Women.*
- *Hydrogen Peroxide - Medical Miracle*
- *Into The Light - Tomorrow's Medicine Today*
- *Lethal Injections - Why Immunizations Don't Work*
- *Painful Dilemma -- Patients In Pain -- People In Prison*
- *Prostate Problems: Safe, Simple Effective Relief*
- *St. Petersburg Nights*
- *Stop Aging Or Slow The Process: Exercise With Oxygen Therapy*
- *The Eagle's Feather*
- *The Joy Of Mature Sex And How To Be A Better Lover...*
- *The Smoker's Paradox: The Health Benefits Of Tobacco*

Introduction

What's a Doctor to Do?

George Bernard Shaw remarked in his book, *The Doctor's Dilemma*, that the same profit motive which assured the manufacture of bread was also at work in the amputation of limbs. Those are pretty harsh words from the old socialist, but he wasn't far from wrong.

The same pattern continues today. Just name a growth industry for the '90s; I'll give you two of the best — soft drinks and drugs. When you think about it, the two aren't very far apart. Both spend millions in glitzy advertising to cajole and con consumers into purchasing useless, mostly harmful products. I'm not just talking about the medicine pitchpersons, like the Tylenol lady, whom you see on TV every night. The "ethical" drug companies (that's what they call themselves because they deal only with doctors and that makes them ethical) now pitch *prescription* drugs to the general public so the patient can say to their doctor: "Hey Doc, why don't we try that new tranquilizer, FEELGOOD. It's more gentle, makes you sleep like a log, and is now recommended by more doctors than brand X in a ratio of 10 to one — I saw it on TV."

What's a doctor to do? Was G.B. Shaw right in his grotesque criticism of the medical profession? The doctor thinks darkly: "If I don't give this guy a FEELGOOD prescription, he's just going to go to another doctor and get it anyway." Scratch, scratch, scratch: "Take one pill Q.I.D. prn to combat consciousness" — another medical triumph (and the doctor's way of saying in Latin, "drop dead").

Americans, barraged with warnings about the dangers of crack and other street drugs, *have more to fear from the medicine they get from their doctor*. Most Americans will not come into contact with crack, but they can get exposed to some lethal stuff, and be completely unaware of it, from their family doctor.

The drug giant Eli Lilly told your doctor that Oraflex was "safer than aspirin" for arthritis. After it killed a lot of people, it was taken off the market. I'm glad you weren't one of the victims — we need all the readers we can get.

The Beecham company wasn't helping our business either. They said that Selacryn was "a first step for high blood pressure." It turned out to be a step to the grave for many patients and was, eventually, removed from the market.

According to Dr. Brian Strom, a leading specialist in pharmaco-epidemiology, 20 percent of all drug therapies cause adverse side effects ranging from nausea to fatal ailments. Side effects put an estimated 1.6 million people in the hospital yearly. *Up to 160,000 of these patients die.* Hospital costs from these disasters amount to $20 billion yearly.

With alarming frequency, drugs cause serious and often fatal side effects that drug makers and the FDA *were unable to identify before the drug was approved.* This was the conclusion of a report from the General Accounting Office (GAO) of your government. Dr. Strom added the following significant observation: "People have this very important misconception that drugs are safe when they are FDA-approved."

Until this GAO study, no one had ever measured how often unidentified serious side effects occurred in new drugs after their release to the public through their doctor. You may find that frightening and hard to believe — so did I.

According to the GAO study, more than half the new drugs approved by the FDA between 1976 and 1985 had serious "post approval" side effects that could lead to hospitalization, disability, or death. And Dr. Strom concluded: "I don't think there is any alternative but to use the first people as guinea pigs."

Recommendation: NEVER allow your doctor to prescribe a new drug for your treatment. Tell *him* to try it first.

Before I go on, I need to say that it would be hypocritical of me, and a disservice to you and the drug industry, not to point out that drugs, when used properly and appropriately, are a great blessing to mankind. If you get bacterial meningitis and don't get the appropriate antibiotic, you are going to die, and that's that. No amount of herbal therapy, touchy-feely love incantations, peroxide, homeopathy, crystals, adjustments, electrotherapy, colonies, vitamin C (or any other vitamin or mineral), magnets, or little black boxes — or a combination of all of the above — will save you.

If you were living in the 19th century and got shot in the stomach, the odds of you living were about one in 100. Today, unless a major blood vessel were to be hit, you would survive 95 percent of the time.

Anesthetics are clearly poisonous and dangerous. The side effects can linger long after the operation and can be permanent. But how would you like to have brain surgery without anesthesia?

Antibiotics, anesthetics, insulin, cortisone to some extent, atropine, epinephrine, anticoagulants, and digitalis have been a boon to mankind when used appropriately. Most of the rest of the *Physicians' Desk Reference* we could do without. Now, having got that off my chest, let's proceed with the drug-bashing.

Compared to this country's major drug companies, the folks at Coke and Pepsi are sweethearts — real humanitarians. When it comes to unscrupulous promotion, bribery, government manipulation, and price gouging, the drug industry tops the bill. Here's the bottom line: America is the drug capital of the world. And I'm not talking about crack and cocaine. I'm speaking of so-called "therapeutic" drugs like Valium, Cortisone, "chemotherapy" drugs, blood pressure pills, anti-cholesterol pills, muscle relaxants (that are nothing but disguised tranquilizers), sleeping pills (that are nothing but variations of Valium), anti-dizzy pills (that don't work), skin creams (that are invariably some form of cortisone — the dermatologists would go out of business without cortisone cream), heart pills that often do more harm than good (and can *kill* you), vasodilators that *don't* dilate your blood vessels but *do* shrink your pocketbook, salves for growing hair, and thousands of copycat drugs made by little companies you never heard of. (But at least the copycats bring down the price.)

The drug situation is about to become much worse. The "animal pharm" in your drug store is about to be greatly expanded. The shelves will soon be stocked with pills for you to buy without a prescription — pills that you were formerly told were too dangerous to take without a doctor's supervision. Now you can forget the doctor and let Angela Lansbury, the druggist, or Doctor Mom be your medical consultant. If you think doctors have been irresponsible in prescribing drugs, wait until you do it on your own for awhile. If one pill is good, wouldn't four be better? If the symptoms get worse after starting your self-medication, shouldn't you double the dose? If product A is good, and B and C cured those folks on TV in about three seconds, why not take all three?

Feldene, an anti-arthritis drug available only by prescription at this time, may be one of the first of the new crop of suddenly-safe drugs. Over 70 deaths have been linked to Feldene.

The FDA is about to throw the public into shark-infested waters. Those sharks are known as "ethical drug companies." We're going to show you, in the pages to follow, how "ethical" they really are.

Physicians from other parts of the world think that American doctors are crazy — and they're right. Americans are drugged virtually to death by greedy drug companies and the narrow vision of the AMA.

What about the FDA — the supposed watchdog of the drug industry? FDA bureaucrats are part of the problem, not the solution. Do they protect the public or just protect their jobs?

The incestuous relationship between drug companies and the FDA is legendary. The level of corruption and collusion is unparalleled. The FDA protects the interests of the major drug companies. That's always been paramount to well-paid FDA officials because they are well taken care of by the drug boys after they finish their "tour" at FDA.

Because of my uncomplimentary remarks about the FDA, government attorneys labeled me "a conspiracy theorist with a very active imagination." *(U.S.A. vs. Vital Health Products, Ltd.)* I was flattered.

Year in and year out, drug companies parade an endless line of new drugs before the FDA; year in and year out the FDA approves these drugs — ignoring negative test data while agency officials end up on the payroll of the very drug companies they are supposed to be monitoring.

But some of the crooks in the FDA have been found out. Four FDA chemists are now making license plates after having been caught taking bribes amounting to thousands of dollars from drug companies making generic drugs. Even the chief of the generic drug division was caught lying about "gratuities" he had received from generic drug companies.

Raju Vegesna, president of American Therapeutics Inc., admitted to paying a $60,000 bribe to an FDA chemist for favorable treatment of his generic drug application. He also bribed an FDA consumer information officer with $20,000 (peanuts to a drug lord like Vegesna) for a peek at the confidential files of a competitor. Vegesna high-tailed it to his native India to escape two years in the cooler. You can rest assured he is a millionaire at your expense and, of course, at the expense of the unlucky patients who may have died from his junk drugs.

K.C. Bae, the Korean owner of Chicago's My-K Laboratories, admitted paying $25,000 to one of your "civil servants" at the FDA. He served a mere three months in jail and paid a measly $25,000 fine. I say measly because he sold the company *and walked away with $20 million.* Makes you wonder how much the judge was paid. Incidentally, Bae was honored as "minority entrepreneur of the year" by the President of the United States. (Sounds like he was a good choice.) I've got an even better one:

Congressional records show that Bolar Pharmaceuticals of New York submitted tablets to the FDA to prove that its product was bio-equivalent to the anti-hypertensive drug, Dyazide. The alleged Bolar tablets turned out to be Dyazide itself that Bolar had purchased at the corner drug store! The FDA was completely fooled by this simple ruse (or bought off?) *which enabled Bolar to generate revenues of over $100 million!*

Recommendation: If you can possibly afford it, don't let the pharmacist substitute a generic drug for the name brand product. In some states, they now substitute without even asking your, or the doctor's, permission. You will pay more for the name brand but, with all the crooked dealing that has been revealed in the FDA, can you afford to take a chance? Of course, with the advent of "socialized" medicine, you will probably be *forced* to take generic drugs.

If the above hasn't convinced you to stick to brand names when you have to take a drug, consider the following horror story.

The generic drug companies are forever mixing up their labels. That's right, the medicine in the bottle isn't what is described on the label. For example, the FDA recently reported that Pharmaceutical Basics of Denver, Colorado, was selling the antidepressant, Desipramine, for the original brand name drug, Norpramin. But the bottles actually contained the anticoagulant, Warfarin. Do you realize how horrific that is? If a patient was taking four to eight Desipramine tablets a day, but the tablets were actually Warfarin, he would almost certainly die of a stroke (cerebral hemorrhage) or from bleeding in the stomach.

In another case that same year, it was found that a muscle relaxant was labeled as the antibiotic Doxycycline. Can you imagine getting a muscle relaxant for your pneumonia? Both of the companies involved in these scandals are infested with crooks. Pharmaceutical Basics has a vice-president in the slammer for giving a $2,000 bribe to an FDA official (maybe they're playing Monopoly together in the same cell) and the other company, Bolar, had its Dyazide diuretic application yanked for presenting a testing sample that was actually their competitor's original product. Other companies have committed this substitution scam, but, in spite of all this crookedness and incompetence, these companies are still in business. Makes you wonder who is *still* getting paid off.

Another case that reveals the FDA's dishonesty and unreliability in the field of generic drugs is the story of Dr. Richard Borison, the chief of psycho-pharmacology at the Augusta, Georgia, Veterans Administration Hospital. Dr. Borison did a study to compare the effectiveness of Thorazine, a tranquilizer, with the generic form of the drug, called Chlorpromazine. Thorazine is the original brand name for the drug.

A group of "aggressive and violent" psychotic patients, who were well-stabilized on Thorazine, were switched to a cheaper, generic form of the drug. The patients rapidly deteriorated and required up to *eight times* as much of the generic medication to gain control. When placed back on Thorazine, they were again controlled at the old dose — a very straightforward result.

But this went contrary to the FDA's doctrine that had ruled generics to be equivalent to brand name drugs. The generic drug companies' bribes of FDA officials had paid off handsomely. The agency's reaction to the report was swift — and lethal to Dr. Borison's career.

The FDA ignored the information in the records, distorted the data, and refused to even listen to Borison and his colleagues. They pronounced him a fraud and, without giving him an opportunity to reply, said his work was fiction. To add to the insult and embarrassment of Dr. Borison, the FDA made these slanderous pronouncements at a meeting of the Generic Manufacturers Association! (Does FDA stand for the "Fraud and Defamation" Administration?)

Several pharmaceutical companies immediately withdrew their research contracts with Borison because, as one told him, "We can't work with you anymore. They're after you on a witch hunt." Three FDA "inspectors" descended upon his laboratory to audit his other studies for drug companies. His career was in a shambles. All the drug companies knew that he was now on the FDA's list of counter-revolutionaries and therefore a non-person.

Dr. Borison plaintively asks: "Can the FDA admit it made a mistake? Can there be other faulty investigations that we don't know about because the FDA has stonewalled inquiry? Can we really say the FDA is adequately protecting the public?"

The answers to these questions are no, yes, and no. And a further answer to the first question is that the FDA didn't make a "mistake." They set out to destroy an investigator who was going against the party line and they succeeded — period.

There are some clear lessons to be learned from this:

(1) Don't mess with any of the communists in the U.S. government, such as the FDA, the USDA, OSHA, and FCC, unless you are prepared to pay the price.

(2) To repeat, if you *must take* a drug, tell your doctor that you don't want a cheap substitute that may have been swept up from the floor of a "laboratory" in Jamaica.

(3) If this principle applies to drugs, it also should apply to nutrients. Don't buy cheap vitamins. Would you buy a bargain-basement parachute?

(4) We need a separation of science and state.

Let me give you another good example of our need for a separation of science and state. The vegetable oil industry has made a lot of false claims about their oils preventing heart attacks. But, for some reason, the Food and Drug Administration never could seem to get around to prosecuting them for misleading the public. The chief prosecutor for the FDA resigned and where do you suppose he went? He became the president of the Institute of Shortening and Edible Oils. Do you suppose he had some idea of where his future lay when, as chief prosecutor for the FDA, he couldn't find the time to prosecute the oil industry for making outrageous claims about vegetable oils and their so-called protective effect against heart attacks?

But the situation is even oilier than that. When the FDA's hired gun quit and joined the "opposition," the oil industry's legal beagle, who had been representing the industry against their now-president, also switched sides and became the chief prosecutor for the FDA!

What about your doctor? Unfortunately, many physicians, although well meaning, are nothing more than pushers for the drug conglomerates. Doctors are literally bombarded with drug company literature proclaiming the newest, greatest miracle pill or procedure.

Doctors are courted by drug company salesmen — given free trips, special gifts, and kickbacks for recommending drugs to their patients. The AMA has finally been embarrassed into taking at least desultory action against the most blatant forms of baksheesh (that's what the Arabs call it) being accepted by its members. But remember, they are taking "action" *against behavior they previously said didn't exist.*

What started as gifts of ballpoint pins, stuffed animals, games, magic tricks, socks, diplomas, nail clippers, note pads containing the company's logo, and other trinkets, has burgeoned into a shameful seduction involving expensive trips to romantic places, such as cruises to the South Pacific, sumptuous dinners, elaborate entertainment, and outright cash bribes, sometimes amounting to thousands of dollars. In 1988, the "ethical" drug industry spent $165 million in "dash" (that's what the Africans call it) to doctors in one form or another — an increase of 400 percent in 15 years.

One drug company offered the doctors "frequent flyer" points for every prescription written for one of their products. (I hope the tickets were on Aeroflot.) The state of

Massachusetts banned this crass commercialization of the doctor-patient relationship and fined the company $195,000. But should that have been necessary?

Don't doctors have any ethics left? Of course all doctors don't succumb to this blatant bribery (certainly not *your* doctor), but many must or the drug companies wouldn't continue to do it and the state wouldn't have to intervene. Maybe the doctors are bringing socialized medicine on themselves. The trouble is, many of them deserve it — but you and I don't, and we'll pay the bill.

Organized medicine should stop worrying about competition from alternative health practitioners, such as chiropractors and homeopaths, and *dean up its own act.* How can doctors expect their patients to have any confidence in their prescriptions or their advice on such life-and-death matters as cancer therapy, if patients are wondering how much money doctors are making because they are suggesting one particular line of therapy as opposed to another?

Chapter 1

A Night at the Opera

A congressional hearing has revealed some very clever promotional methods by the drug companies designed to appear "scientific" but which are nothing but payoffs. "A Night at the Opera" was one of the cleverest.

Abbott Laboratories purchased a night at the opera for psychiatrists attending a medical meeting in New York. The company had arranged for singers to perform a recital of "the great neurotic episodes" from opera. The printed program given to the docs described each condition, advertised the company's drug, the tranquilizer, Tranxene, and *conferred credits for medical education* to the doctors who attended this "scientific" session. (Did they give the wives a free sample of Tranxene? A missed opportunity if they didn't: "A survey shows that more psychiatrists' wives use Tranxene than any other....")

You'll have to admit this opera thing was quite a creative scam — give credit where credit is due. Tranxene rapidly became the leading brain-shrinking drug used by psychiatrists, even though many of the clinical indications for the drug suggested by the company *had absolutely no scientific backing.* The doctors must have really liked the opera. (And, anyway, who ever said psychiatrists were scientific?)

The manipulation of doctors by drug companies has gone high-tech. A front organization for a group of ten of the biggest drug companies, called Physicians Computer Network, will install a $35,000 office computer system, *absolutely free* to the doctor. Don't you think doctors would be smart enough to realize that the drug giants are not doing this out of the goodness of their stone hearts?

Drug salesmen swarm over doctors in private practice like ants on a rotten carcass. The biggies, like Lilly, Roche and Bristol, wanted to get a leg up on the little guys. Some marketeers got the brilliant idea of worming their way into the doctor's computer system by donating the expensive equipment for the exchange of information about the doctor's prescribing habits. That way they will know if he wanders from the fold and prescribes a *verboten* product.

And the doctor is expected to do more: He must agree to watch regular "command performances" on video of the companies' drug ads and he must, to justify their expensive bribe, agree to watch 32 promotional messages a month and "answer one clinically oriented question per message." (This keeps him honest.)

So the companies not only have a monitor on his prescribing habits (and whatever else may be in the computer), but they also have control of his brain. If he starts prescribing the wrong drug, they simply sit him down and show him the correct drug and have him answer a "clinical" question about that drug —- just to be sure he got the message. Have you ever heard of anything so disgusting?

I recently received a questionnaire from a "research group" inquiring into my prescription habits. Enclosed was a check for $5 which, they said, was not for my time but was just a friendly gesture, or something like that. I kept their five bucks and threw their questionnaire in the waste basket. If more doctors would do that, it might stop all this prying and bribing.

Connaught Laboratories had a great thing going to promote the sale of vaccines. You probably thought that vaccines were given to people on the basis of some medical need. Not necessarily. With the VIP Program (very important purchaser), the more the doc stuck his patients with vaccines, the more VCRs, video cameras, computers, and "medical education" programs he would receive — just like green stamps, only it's *your* money (and maybe your health) paying for the stamps.

After being threatened with an anti-kickback prosecution by the Department of Health and Human Services, Connaught dropped the program.

Chapter 2
Tagamet: The Start of It All

The drug industry used to think that the demand for drugs was inelastic, like burial plots or dentures. There are only so many patients with a certain disease and once you fill that demand, the profit curve will level off. But all that changed with the introduction of Tagamet. The manufacturer produced a flood of publicity that was so effective that people were asking their doctors for the drug *before it was even available.* The other pharmaceutical companies took note and realized they had a new tool for greatly expanding the market for a particular drug. Beyond what the *doctor* thought was best for the patient, they could now appeal to what the *patient* thought was best for the patient. A little oiling of the doctor, such as the brilliant opera ploy, would perhaps convince the doctor that maybe the patient really *does* know best. After all, the drugs are safe, aren't they?

Let's take a look at Tagamet, the one that started this drug-feeding frenzy — then we'll resume the payola story. Tagamet helps ulcers and gives rapid relief of the symptoms of duodenal and gastric ulcers; there's no doubt about that. Sure, it can cause depression, mental confusion, anxiety, hallucinations, disorientation, swelling of the breasts, impotence, fever, heart irregularities, rash, and kidney disease but, hey, we're talking real live relief from stomach pain here. The odds are you won't get any of the above harmful side effects from Tagamet anyway, so don't get an ulcer worrying about it.

But there is one little item you need to know about Tagamet that could save your life. And if your doctor doesn't read the *Wall Street Journal,* he may not have heard of it. If you are on Tagamet and you are exposed to pesticides in your yard, say, while mowing the lawn, you may develop an epilepsy-like disease, brain tumor symptoms, cancer, and multiple sclerosis all rolled into one. You may not die, but you'll probably wish that you were dead.

That's what happened to Thomas Latimer, age 36, as reported in the *Wall Street Journal* of October 14, 1991. He was on a standard dose of Tagamet and, after *only one hour* of exposure to lawn pesticide, while mowing his lawn, his life turned into a living hell. He developed all of the above symptoms and went from a successful petroleum engineer to a near-basket case.

What happened is clear. Tagamet is well known to interfere with the breakdown of other chemicals. If you are on an anticoagulant, for instance, Tagamet may prevent the drug from being broken down in the liver and you can bleed to death due to an overdose. You can also suffer an "internal overdose" if you are taking a diuretic, a tranquilizer, a heart drug, Valium, or almost anything else in conjunction with Tagamet. Mr. Latimer received a dose of organophosphate pesticide that would not ordinarily harm a healthy 36-year-old man. But the Tagamet blocked the metabolism of the chemical in the liver and, according to many experts, this caused the poison to accumulate in tissues through his body. According to the experts, it will stay in his fat cells "indefinitely."

Alfredo A. Sadun, professor of neurosurgery at the University of California, says taking a medication like Tagamet "can make a person 100 to 1,000 times more sensitive to organophosphate poisoning."

The government admits that it has absolutely no idea of how to test for these lethal interactions between drugs like Tagamet and the pesticides on your lawn. The drug companies are not required to do more than essentially irrelevant tests on mice. You are on your own.

The drug interaction phenomenon is quite common but patients are unaware of it and doctors tend to ignore it. For instance, if you are taking Seldane for an allergy and you are also prescribed Nizoral for Candida or some other fungal infection, you can drop dead from a fatal heart spasm (cardiac arrhythmia). If you are taking Seldane from your allergist and then you get an infection for which your family doctor prescribes the antibiotic, Erythromycin, you may have the same result: death from a heart spasm.

An even more common interaction that can have deadly consequences is that of Tylenol and the anticoagulant, Coumadin. Tylenol blocks the destruction of Coumadin in the liver, just like the Tagamet-pesticide interaction, and you can bleed to death from an excess of the Coumadin.

So, as you can see, the *2,500 possible side effects* of drugs are not your-only problem. With the interaction problem, 25,000 is a more realistic estimate of the possible jams you can get into.

Recommendation: If you are on multiple drugs, including the nostrums sold in the drugstore, and your doctor can't tell you what to expect from the combination (and he probably can't), the only way to protect yourself is to purchase the computer disc called Drug Interactions and Side Effects from the people who publish the *Physicians Desk Reference* (800-232-7379). It will cost you $235 so maybe you can talk your library into purchasing it.

Chapter 3
Payola and Prostitution

And now back to our payola story.

Sometimes the bribes given to doctors are absolutely obscene. Take the case of a Florida doctor who was offered $1,200 by Roche Laboratories as a "grant-in-aid" (is that the way the drug industry spells "baksheesh"?) to do a clinical study on a drug called Rocephin. The study would take about four minutes per patient and the compensation factored out to $900 per hour. The $1,200 is peanuts to Roche. They make $11,400 on 20 patients treated for only 10 days.

At the congressional hearing mentioned above, a pharmacist told of the undue influence the drug companies have on the dispensing of medicines in the hospital. Some hospitals, he reported, have been threatened with withdrawal of "research support" if the hospital's pharmacy doesn't give the company's products the support they think they deserve. The witness, Arthur Zoloth, was clearly disturbed by what he had seen in the medical "industry": "I find this pervasive presence of the drug companies in the medical system to be repugnant. Thus we see on the one hand, physicians making very nice incomes, accepting all sorts of largess from pharmaceutical companies, including free trips, free educational courses, various handouts and gifts, and on the other hand, many patients are struggling to afford essential medications which frequently cost over a $100 a month apiece. I find this ethically and professionally distasteful."

When I was practicing in Atlanta, the neighborhood was *swarming* with drug salesmen (and women) but none *ever* came to my office — no free ballpoints, no dinners at the Ritz-Carlton. They never even asked *me* to go on a Caribbean cruise. The drug salesmen have a network and the word quickly goes out as to which doctors are "anti-drug."

Being black-balled by the sleaze brigade is a backhanded compliment, but I always wondered something about those guys I could never confirm. Do the drug companies supply them with "companions" for their little meetings? Seems to be an obvious question, since prostitutes speak a common language.

Busy doctors don't have the time personally to research the efficacy of each new drug. A patient is ill; a new drug promises relief; the doctor prescribes it. It's a never-ending circle that only helps to push this country further into the hands of the drug company-FDA-AMA cartel.

Most doctors are ignorant of the limitations of drug therapy or they don't want to admit, even to themselves, that most of the drugs they prescribe do very little, do nothing, or do harm to the patient. Many of the drugs act as "negative placebos," i.e., there are side effects to the prescription and so the patient thinks he must be getting some good it. "It must be working because I feel so lousy," he says to himself.

The Powerful Placebo Effect

The placebo is extremely important and is understood by patients only superficially. In fact, it's understood by doctors and drug researchers only superficially. The double-blind study, in which one group of patients receives the experimental drug and the other a placebo (and neither the patient nor the doctor is supposed to know which are which) is ridiculous, pointless, and fraught with danger, if you just look at the method realistically.

The placebo effect, where one thinks he is better because of a strong suggestibility factor, is extremely powerful. For example, a patient of mine had atrial fibrillation and was told by a cardiologist that there was a good chance that the heart flutter would go away if he would stop drinking alcohol. He quit his nightly (four-finger) highball, wine with dinner (two four-ounce glasses), and after-dinner Bristol Creme. His fibrillation went away immediately and he didn't have the slightest twitch from his heart for two weeks — a miracle. But then it returned and was worse than before. So he had experienced a powerful placebo effect *without taking any medicine at all.* Just the mere suggestion had given him two weeks completely symptom-free.

With a drug, the placebo effect is *even stronger* than with the placebo itself, because the patient, unless he is a moron, usually knows he is on a drug and not a starch pill, because of the almost inevitable side effects of the drug. If there is no side effect, then it is not an effective drug, because the desired therapeutic effect is a side effect, itself. It just happens to be a side effect that you want, such as lowering the blood pressure.

If the patient on the blood pressure-lowering medication feels tiredness, dizziness, impotence, or any other of the dozens of side effects that he can get from the medication, then the therapeutic effect will be reinforced by the placebo effect and the drug will appear, at least for a while, to be *vastly superior* to the placebo. But, as the placebo effect wears off, the pill will lose its effectiveness, and the doctor will be puzzled as to why.

This phenomenon, which I call the symptom-enhanced placebo effect (SEPE), explains why so many drugs are put on the market and, in a few years, just fade away into that vast graveyard of wonder drugs, separated from their placebo cover. What ever happened to Maxitate, Atromid, Mellaril, Dexedrine, Darvon, and Salutensin? If you were to look in a *Physicians' Desk Reference* of 20 years ago, you would be surprised at how many dead wonder drugs are there. They are all in the SEPE graveyard.

Remember that the double-blind, placebo-controlled study is the way that all drugs make their way to your medicine cabinet. But the double-blind is almost always a scientific farce. The patient will become aware of side effects. He will report these to his doctor. The doctor now knows that the patient is on the drug and not the placebo. The game is up. At this point neither the patient nor the doctor is blind and they both realize that it is now a charade. Such is the status of drug science.

If you think the FDA and/or your doctor is protecting you from dangerous drugs, you could be fatally mistaken. There's only one solution: You must protect yourself. You must be cautious, skeptical, and well-informed when it comes to drug use.

That's the purpose of this book — to give you the information you need to make wise decisions concerning the drugs you take. Trusting and naive patients are the driving force behind drug company profits and prescription-happy physicians. To stop the vicious circle you must learn for yourself the value and dangers of legal drugs. And you must resist the idiotic philosophy, so rampant in this country, that a miracle pill can cure anything that ails you. Don't look to your doctor as a drug-giver. He should be giving you treatment, not drugs.

Most common health problems are not dangerous. Sure, they're annoying, but if left alone they'll go away. But add drugs to the formula and you run the greater risk of encountering serious, sometimes fatal, side effects. And if you don't suffer from taking useless drugs, your wallet certainly will.

Chapter 4

Drugs and the Common Cold

A recent study from Johns Hopkins University confirms what I have been telling anxious mothers for 25 years: If your child has a cold, give him plenty of attention, a little chicken soup — and maybe a little ice cream. *Don't* give him aspirin, decongestants, antihistamines, sedatives, Tylenol and, most importantly, *don't give him antibiotics.* If the kid gets *really* sick, *you* can tell (you're his mother aren't you?) and then take him to the doctor. I'm not saying pediatricians aren't necessary (I'm glad *I* don't have to take care of all those screaming, sniveling, coughing, squirming little monst... excuse me, precious and adorable children), but the doctor's services are definitely overused by the average American mom.

In the study, the researchers found *no difference* in the recovery rate between children receiving medication (usually a combination of expectorant for cough and an antihistamine which acts as a sedative), a placebo — or nothing. More than half the children were better in two days no matter what was done.

Doctors routinely prescribe some type of medication because they think it will help or (in most cases) because they feel they have to placate the mother into feeling that "something was done." (How else can you justify a $50 fee?) If you are a ghetto parent the doctor has to be more careful and watch a little more closely because your child is probably malnourished, thus immune-deficient and more susceptible to *real* disease. But, ironically, these are the children who get the least expert care and less attention. Life isn't fair and there isn't much you can do about it. But the best way to get a fair deal for *your* child is to give him as few drugs as possible.

What to do:

    (1)   Remain calm. (Easy for me to say — right?)

(2)   Is the child eating well? If so, he isn't very sick.
(3)   What is his temperature? If it's below 101° F, you're O.K.
(4)   If the temperature is 101° F in the *morning*, that's fairly high.
(5)   If the doctor wants to give your child antibiotics, refuse them until he does a blood count. When the count comes back, if you want to sound learned, ask him: "Well, doctor, is the white count elevated and is there a shift to the left?" More than likely he will respond: "Well, no, it is not elevated and there is a relative lymphocytosis." You reply: "Ah yes, then antibiotics are not indicated as this is undoubtedly a viral infection." To which he replies: "Hmm, well, that's true so why don't we just give him a little expectorant-antihistamine to tide him over?"

Now you have another problem. You just learned above that doctors at Johns Hopkins University found these drugs are ineffective for the treatment of colds. After you point this out to him, your relationship will have become rather strained. If you like the guy, and want him when a *real* emergency comes up, just take the piece of paper he hands you and *don't* get it filled.

(6)   Even if the child has had febrile convulsions in the past, there is no reason to panic. Just keep him cool with towels that are room temperature. Febrile convulsions don't affect the brain and these kids grow up normal just like the rest of us. (I had a *lot* of fever convulsions when I was a child and look how smart I am.)
(7)   Does he have a stiff neck? If he does, *now* it's time to panic. You're probably wrong, and he probably doesn't have meningitis, but when you call the doctor and say "He has a stiff neck," I'll guarantee he'll beat you to the hospital.

Adults with Colds

What about adults with colds? I can't think of many things as exploitative as the television commercials for cold remedies.

They are all essentially identical, but the advertising during the flu season is frenetic and constant. Flu is by far the most costly disease in the United States. Yet, none of the remedies shorten the disease by as much as one hour and might even prolong it.

The medicine men of the old west were rank amateurs compared to today's TV snake oil salesmen. The woman on TV rubs her temples, furrows her brow and peers into the camera: "Only Dristan Sinus combines the leading decongestant with the modern pain-reliever, ibuprofen." A baldfaced lie. American Home Products, the makers of Dristan Sinus, also sells CoAdvil which has the same ingredients and the same doses as their other cold nostrum. But they are different in the minds of the average gullible consumer. Dristan Sinus is for sinus headaches and CoAdvil is for colds. The TV commercials will keep you straight.

Johnson and Johnson, one of those "ethical" drug companies, sells Tylenol Cold and Tylenol Cold and Flu. Now if you had a cold and the flu (don't ask me how you make that diagnosis — maybe Dr. Mom knows) then you wouldn't want to just take Tylenol Cold, would you? Well, maybe you would — the products are identical.

The drug company Schering-Plough markets Drixoral Plus and Drixoral Sinus and, although they are almost identical, one of them is described as "The only 12-hour sinus medicine." Note I said almost identical — Drixoral sinus pills are yellow and Drixoral Plus tablets are green. Drixoral Plus is for pain and fever. Drixoral Sinus is for sinus.

The four major ingredients in all the cold nostrums, from Contac to Co-Tylenol, are analgesic/antipyretic, anti-tussive, antihistamine and decongestant.

The analgesic/antipyretic (pain/temperature-lowering) is always aspirin, Tylenol or a combination of both. They may help you to sleep if you are having the "aches and pains" they are always preaching about on TV. They will not shorten the disease. Stop taking them after the first or second day of your cold. The elevated temperature needs no treatment and is part of the body's defense mechanism.

There is only one anti-tussive (cough suppressant) medication that you can get without a prescription and that's Dextromethorphan. Many of the cold remedies contain it. But, do you want to depress your cough? The cough mechanism helps you expectorate all the gook in your bronchial tubes. If it collects there, you may get pneumonia; and prolonged suppression of the cough reflex can lead to bronchiectasis — pus pockets in the lungs, something you definitely don't want. It's OK to take a little dextromethorphan at bed time to suppress the cough enough so that you can get some rest. But discontinue it as soon as the cough abates. Codeine is a far better cough suppressant but it's not available without a prescription and you may not be willing to fork out $50 for the doctor visit plus $5 more for the prescription. (I wouldn't.)

Many smokers come to me complaining that they had the flu but the cough won't go away. If they don't understand the obvious problem, what am I supposed to say? For what it's worth, I say, "Quit smoking." It's never well-received.

The decongestant in most of these remedies is phenylpropanolamine. A decongestant is supposed to do just that: decongest you. But taken by mouth they are essentially worthless and they can keep you awake because they are basically a form of speed. A far better choice for clearing up your nose so that you can breathe and sleep is Afrin spray. Afrin really works and the effect will last all night for most people. It's great stuff when used appropriately. Give yourself a squirt in each nostril *but only at bed time* — you can become dependant on it if you use it habitually. Don't use it full strength in small children — in fact, do consult your doctor about that.

The antihistamine in cold products is a waste of money and serves no useful purpose other than making you drowsy. Products which contain it should not be taken during the day if you need to stay alert. It's useful in allergies, but its inclusion in cold medication is totally irrational.

Certain of the cold products deserve special mention:

- *Contac* contains a decongestant and an antihistamine — it is an expensive and worthless product.

- *Coricidin* is a combination of an antihistamine and Tylenol. Just buy Tylenol (acetaminophen) if you want something for pain and don't waste your money on the antihistamine.

- *Co-Tylenol* is a terrible and expensive shotgun combination that should be avoided. It has many peers.

- *Dristan* is like the other combination cold drugs, illogical. But even worse, the ingredients vary depending on which of the products called Dristan that you purchase. The capsules, tablets, nasal spray, and "nighttime liquid" are *all different chemicals* but they are all called Dristan. Which one of them is for you? None of them.

- *Robitussin* is Dr. Mom's favorite for her kiddies and her dopey husband. (Why are husbands always depicted as morons in the TV commercials?) The actress who plays everybody's young mother is selling you a bill of drug-tainted goods. The commercial strongly implies that Robitussin cures colds. (It doesn't — nothing does.) The product should be labeled as knock-out drops. Your Uncle Harry, the one with the W.C. Fields red nose, would love Robitussin — *it's 20-proof alcohol.* Does Dr. Mom serve it to her kids straight or on the rocks? This expensive mix contains an antihistamine which, along with the 20-proof alcohol, is bound to put your kids into a nice coma. The company would call it sleep. I call it coma. (Try to wake them up — see what I mean?) Mom should have her medical license revoked for pushing dope on minors.

- *Nyquil Cold Medicine* is another mixture of drugs and booze that goes head-to-head with Robitussin. Nyquil is *50-proof* alcohol so you definitely want to give it to Uncle Harry, not your kids.

- *Excedrin* is another illogical shotgun that contains three different drugs for pain. Why subject yourself to the side effects of three different drugs when one will do? It is heavily promoted during the flu season in the hope that there will be an unconscious linking of Excedrin with the cure of flu. The ploy works fabulously well, the product doesn't.

Chapter 5
Painkillers

This report would not be complete without some remarks about America's number one "nutrient": painkillers. This group includes such "staples" as aspirin, Tylenol, and Darvon.

Let's dispense with Darvon (propoxyphene) first. It is, in my opinion, a worthless analgesic for one simple reason: It doesn't work. It is now sold in combination with acetaminophen (Tylenol) under the name of Darvocet. The company had to do *something* once they realized that Darvon alone was about as useful for pain as saltpeter. Darvon (propoxyphene) can cause serious kidney disease and has addiction potential, whereas aspirin and Tylenol do not. Interestingly, Darvon overdose is quite similar clinically to overdose with morphine (but morphine is a lot more fun). Avoid Darvon. It should be given the heave-ho into the SEPE cemetery.

Aspirin is *número uno* — Americans consume *15 tons* of aspirin every day, 19 *billion* tablets per year. What size container do you suppose it would take to hold 19 billion aspirin tablets — the Rose Bowl maybe?

And it's not just America. Aspirin is *in* — worldwide. An aspirin promotion group called the Aspirin Foundation boasts that the chemical "probably has been taken, at one time or another, by almost every human being on earth."

Wishful thinking perhaps, but the worldwide consumption is enormous. The British take it in a powder; the Italians take an effervescent, champagne-like mix; the French take it rectally, and the Thailanders put it in their tea. Worldwide, chemical companies produce *90 billion* aspirin tablets a year.

Aspirin and Heart Attack: Dangerous BUNK!

The sensational report on aspirin, reported below, really got my attention. Just think, a 47 percent reduction in the incidence of heart attack among men taking aspirin — wow! I dashed to the medicine cabinet to take my aspirin, hoping that I wasn't too late to save my hypochondriacal soul. While pouring the fluoridated, chlorinated, aluminized water from the kitchen sink, I read some of the fine print in the report. It said that when deaths from all causes were considered, there was no difference in mortality rates between men taking the aspirin and those not taking it.

Since death from a massive heart attack is probably the very best way to depart this earth, and since my chances of dying would be the same with or without the aspirin, and having a natural aversion to drugs, I cleverly decided to put the aspirin bottle back in the medicine cabinet to await my next headache.

Did you ever think you would see the day when Americans by the millions would be popping aspirin for their health? Do all these people really have an aspirin deficiency? Did God forget to put aspirin in our food? Will an aspirin a day really keep the doctor away?

I assume that you would say no to all of the above, because it doesn't make any sense to take a chemical as if it were a vitamin. But it took the British to figure out how this madness came about.

The much-promoted Physicians' Health Study "proving" that taking aspirin regularly will prevent heart attacks, didn't use just aspirin, but aspirin *plus magnesium* in the form of Bufferin.

Research done years ago proved that magnesium protects the heart. It dilates blood vessels, aids in the absorption of potassium into cells (which will prevent heartbeat irregularities), acts as an anticoagulant (blood thinner), and keeps the blood cells from sticking together (thrombosis). Autopsies of the heart muscle following death by heart attack almost always reveal that the heart muscle is deficient in magnesium.

I have had hundreds of patients on magnesium for over ten years. We just don't see many heart attacks among patients who stick with it.

So, it turns out, the doctors and their patients have been conned again by the group that has been leading them around by the nose for 75 years — the pharmaceutical industry. A British study using *only* aspirin revealed that aspirin had absolutely nothing to do with lowering the incidence of heart attacks. The American study was so flawed that you can't help but wonder if the aspirin industry financed it. The subjects for the study were white, male, mostly non-smoking doctors who were not monitored and who reported their condition by letter — what I call post office research. The study used an extremely healthy group with only *one-eighth* the death rate of the general population.

But even with such a healthy group, the study results had some ominous overtones. That's the part the aspirin companies don't want you to know about. Though heart attacks were relatively rare among the group, strokes and sudden death from other causes were more common among the aspirin group compared to the placebo group.

The claim for reduction in heart attacks among the aspirin group was 47 percent. But the small print (*very* small print) in the report said that when death from all causes was considered, there was *no difference* in the mortality rates of the two groups. Thus death from other causes cancelled out the benefits that the magnesium had conferred on the aspirin-taking group.

Every time you take an aspirin you bleed a little into your gut. A microscope will show every time that the bowel movement of someone on daily aspirin contains blood. If it's happening in your gut, how do you know it's not happening in your brain? How many strokes are precipitated by chronic aspirin intake? How many fatal hemorrhages of the brain, spleen, liver, intestine or lung occur after an automobile accident because the blood was thinned with aspirin? Nobody knows and nobody is checking.

I've never heard anyone claim that aspirin is addicting, but a Mayo Clinic report makes you wonder. They reported on five cases of chronic duodenal ulcer caused by the habitual use of aspirin. The patients all had to undergo surgery for bleeding from the duodenum secondary to their aspirin abuse. In every case, the patients denied that they took aspirin. But blood tests for aspirin revealed "therapeutic levels" in all of them.

In spite of going through the trauma of surgery, all of them had a repeat episode of bleeding ulcer. Again, they all repeatedly denied taking aspirin. But blood tests again revealed high levels of aspirin in every single case.

At this point the surgeons threw up their hands and referred the patients to a psychiatrist. It's possible that some of these people really *didn't* know they were taking aspirin because it travels under so many aliases: Doan's Pills, Excedrin, Midol, salicylic acid, sodium salicylate, Vanquish, Darvon Compound-65 and many, many more.

At any rate, there are many natural ways to protect yourself from heart attack without enriching the Bayer company:

- *Magnesium,* as mentioned above, is absolutely essential for a healthy heart and should be given credit for the beneficial results obtained in the aspirin study.
- *Salmon oil* contains a strong platelet anti-sticking agent called eicosapentaenoic acid (as long as you can pronounce salmon oil, don't worry about it). Olive oil is also excellent for your heart.
- *Garlic* also tends to block the clotting mechanism.
- *Vitamin B-6* stops platelet aggregation.
- *Niacin* is a well-known anti-atherosclerotic (hardening of the arteries) agent.
- *Vitamin C* is an important factor in prostaglandin production and hence is cardio-protective.
- *Vitamin E* is also important in the production of prostaglandins.
- *Bromelin* reduces platelet stickiness.
- *Zinc* is a necessary catalyst in certain metabolic processes essential to the health of your arteries.
- *Vitamin B-6,* mentioned earlier, also converts the highly atherogenic (artery hardening) homocystine from over-

cooked meat to cystathionine and thus prevents it from damaging your arteries.

- *Folic acid* neutralizes the atherogenic xanthine oxidase found in homogenized milk.
- *Carnitine* and *taurine,* two of the amino acids considered non-essential by most dieticians, are absolutely essential for a healthy heart.

It is impossible to say exactly how much of these various nutrients you should take to protect your heart. The studies haven't been done because the research institutions aren't interested. Even if they were interested, what pharmaceutical company or government agency is going to supply the funds? Take one or two of the standard pills or capsules of each of the nutrients mentioned. Don't take massive doses of any of them. You can definitely overdo a good thing.

A few years ago, I was in Nashville, Tennessee attending a medical conference with a colleague. While at dinner he developed severe chest pain, was rushed to the university hospital, and was found to have suffered a heart attack.

At the emergency room, everyone was very casual and nothing was done other than the starting of an intravenous drip. The first few hours are very critical for the heart attack victim, as ventricular fibrillation can occur, which is often fatal — even in the hospital setting. Intravenous magnesium should have been the first order of business but it was not administered. Of all the hundreds of agents they use in hospitals, magnesium is one of the most important — and the least used.

Fortunately, my friend did not fibrillate, went to bypass surgery, and survived it.

I was visiting him the following day when a nurse came in to give him his vital medicine — an aspirin tablet! She stood there and watched him take it with a glass of water. Such is the reverence felt for this drug in today's university hospitals.

In addition to the reports showing aspirin has no preventive effect on heart attacks, new reports show that aspirin may cause cancer. Another study by California researchers, reported in the British Medical Journal, revealed that older men and women who take aspirin every day almost double their chances of developing ischemic heart disease — *the very thing that aspirin is supposed to prevent!*

Lawrence Garfinkel, Vice President for Epidemiology at the American Cancer Society said, "It would give one pause about using aspirin routinely to prevent an initial heart attack. This is going to be very confusing to the public." The report concluded: "Our study would not recommend that these people routinely consume aspirin."

Leo Dropperman started taking aspirin to prevent a second heart attack, as advised by his doctor and the TV commercials. But when he read that daily doses of aspirin could increase his chances of getting a hemorrhagic stroke, he quit. "I'd much rather have a heart attack than a stroke," said the Tennessee psychologist. "I'm very vain about my brain."

It's even worse than that, Leo. The British report mentioned earlier found that the aspirin wouldn't prevent your heart attack in the first place. And the California study goes even further in suggesting that daily aspirin use may actually *increase* the odds of having a heart attack, as well as give you colon or kidney cancer.

On receiving these unflattering reports, the aspirin companies quickly folded their aspirin-for-your-heart show. Sterling Drug (Eastman Kodak) pulled its commercial depicting the Bayer aspirin logo over a pulsating heart monitor and substituted the old line: "The wonder drug doctors themselves take more often for pain." (Well, who doesn't take aspirin?) Bristol-Myers went even more low-tech and dragged out medical expert Angela Lansbury to say: "A cup of tea and a couple of Bufferin allow me to do the things I want to do." That's vague enough.

Sterling, ever wanting to help you, introduced a calendar pack so you won't forget your daily aspirin. For what? Because that aspirin a day "will allow you to do the things you want to do." Wouldn't it be great if that were really true?

People don't know whom to believe anymore. Can you trust the FDA? In December, 1984, the FDA recommended allowing drug companies to promote the use of aspirin for reducing the chances of a second heart attack.

Can you trust the medical journals? In 1988, the *New England Journal of Medicine* came out for an aspirin every other day to reduce the risk of a heart attack. Is it coincidental that the drug companies have been able to get their slimy fingers into the *New England Journal of Medicine* with multi-million-dollar contracts?

Can you trust the medical advice given by the likes of Angela Lansbury? I didn't know she was a scientist. I thought she was a crime expert.

For low-grade pain, aspirin is the drug of choice. It is also the drug of first choice, if natural remedies don't work, for rheumatoid arthritis. This particular report is not about natural remedies but I must tell you this: A complete fast will often help arthritis dramatically. Food allergy seems to play a part with some people.

Various brands of aspirin vary widely in price. You can pay a lot or you can pay a little. Most of it is made by the drug giant, Bayer, so if expensive Bayer aspirin makes you feel better than cheap Bayer aspirin, then go for it.

Stay away from Aspergum, the aspirin-containing chewing gum. This is a silly creation comparable to smearing digoxin on your chest for heart failure or antibiotic on your belly for an appendicitis. Applying aspirin to an inflamed throat is completely irrational. Aspirin is not an anesthetic and applying it to the throat, assuming that any of it got there in the first place (it goes down the *esophagus*, not the throat) would only make the inflammation worse due to the acidity of the aspirin.

Aspirin interacts with many drugs and so, before mixing aspirin with other medications, check your *Physicians' Desk Reference.* It could save you a lot of grief. Incidentally, you can purchase the PDR at most major book stores.

Tylenol Tales

Tylenol (acetaminophen), with the help of the Tylenol lady on TV, has taken a big chunk of the pain market away from aspirin. Like aspirin, it is used for pain and fever reduction. I don't think it is as effective as aspirin, but the Tylenol lady is more convincing than I and, besides, she has national television. Tylenol (and Datril, Tempra, Anacin-3, and Liquiprin) has some advantages (and disadvantages) over aspirin:

- It doesn't cause intestinal bleeding.
- Not being in the same family of drugs as aspirin, it can be used when a person has aspirin allergy.
- It doesn't thin the blood like aspirin and so can be used by hemophiliacs and after surgery.
- Stomach upset is not as likely to occur as with aspirin. The downside of acetaminophen:
- It is worthless for rheumatoid arthritis. It is not an effective anti-inflammatory agent.
- It can cause severe liver damage (after all, it *is* a coal tar chemical).
- An allergic skin rash may occur.
- It doesn't work for reducing fever, no matter what the Tylenol lady says on TV.

Now there is serious doubt as to whether aspirin and acetaminophen (Tylenol) should be used at all in children with viral illnesses such as chicken pox, measles, the common cold and flu (which is really nothing but a very bad cold). According to a group of Baltimore researchers, these "harmless" drugs actually prolong the symptoms and so should be used, at most, only at night to help the patient sleep — one dose and that's it.

They did their research on a group of 68 children with chicken pox, which is caused by the varicella-zoster virus. They were testing the effectiveness of Tylenol and found that those children given Tylenol had no significant reduction in temperature and their rash lasted longer than children given a placebo.

One more caveat about aspirin and acetaminophen: In children, they can cause a life-threatening condition called

Reye's syndrome. The disease causes a swelling of the brain and malfunction of the liver.

Many food additives can cause serious and even fatal reactions. Among these are tartrazine, sulfites, and lanolin. Symptoms may include severe wheezing, purple blotches on the skin, itching, rapid heart rate, flushing, and blurred vision. An incomprehensible situation has developed in the Food and Drug Administration. The additive problem is clearly recognized, so the FDA requires food companies to put on the product label all the additives in a given product. *But the same additives can be put in pharmaceuticals without any warning to the public.* So if you have a drug reaction, it may not be the drug at all but the additives. Doctors rarely consider this.

Chapter 6
Drug Side Effects Can Be Serious

A recent report by the Health Research Group of the consumer organization, Public Citizen, reveals some sobering statistics about the side effects of what the FDA labels as "safe and effective" drugs.

- Each year 61,000 older Americans develop drug-induced parkinsonism.

- 32,000 hip fractures are caused by drug-induced falls.

- 163,000 Americans develop drug-induced memory loss or impaired thinking.

- More than 243,000 over the age of 55 are hospitalized each year because of adverse drug reactions.

- More than 2 million older Americans are addicted to minor tranquilizers and/or sleeping pills.

As you can see, prescription drugs can raise havoc in many ways. In fact, adverse reactions and addiction are all too common, especially in people over age 50. And often the result is death, but the death certificate may read "heart attack" or "stroke" because autopsies are seldom done on the elderly. *In other words, no one knows what millions of these older people actually die from.*

Take the case of a 52-year-old-woman who was having some dental work done. She was given a supposedly safe sedative — one that would calm her but keep her conscious while the dentist performed his work. She didn't remain conscious; she died. Fortunately, this sort of tragedy is not common, but I relate the case to make two points: (1) You don't really have to be old to have a fatal reaction to a drug and (2) Drugs can *never* be assumed to be entirely safe.

You know I'm not a fan of the World Health Organization (WHO), but occasionally even bureaucrats mess up and
get things right (even a blind pig can find an acorn once in a
while). Reporting on the number of fatalities and adverse reactions suffered by normally healthy adults, WHO said,
"Quite often, the history and clinical examination of patients
with side-effects reveal that no valid indication for the drug
has been present."

Cutting through the bureaucratic double-speak, WHO is
basically saying that there was no reason to give patients the
drugs. If you take WHO's thinking a step further, there can be
only one conclusion: "Quite often," as WHO put it, people are
given too many drugs for problems which could be better
treated with non-drug therapy.

In this country, and to a lesser degree the countries of
Western Europe, doctors use drugs to treat the natural
physical and psychological changes associated with aging.
We're trying to ward off the aging process by using
dangerous drugs that actually may speed the process. That's
not good medicine; it's not even good sense.

Doctors love to prescribe pills for older Americans, and
older Americans love getting them. People over 60 make up
about 15 percent of this country's population. They use 40
percent of the prescription drugs — more than 650 million
prescriptions each year. That's a lot of pills, and a lot of
money in the pockets of the drug company cartels. A
conservative estimate is that more than 60 percent of those
prescriptions are either unnecessary inappropriate, or entirely
too risky for the patient to use.

And the older you get, the worse it gets. More than 65
percent of people over the age of 65 take a cardiovascular
drug for high blood pressure or other related diseases. There's
no doubt that many of these elderly people need a drug for
the heart — in cases of heart failure, for instance — but most
of them would be better off without medicine for high blood
pressure. I fact, they may have their lives shortened by the
medication.

More than 33 percent of this age group also take what
called a psychotropic drug — a tranquilizer, a "mood

elevator" or a sedative. These drugs are often used in nursing homes and psychiatric hospitals as a "warehousing" tool to keep the patients quiet and easily manageable. They are for the benefit of the staff not the patients. Elderly patients may be diagnosed as having Alzheimer's disease when their real problem is actually overdosage with psychotropic drugs. It's not at all uncommon for an alert relative to insist that all medications of a depressing nature be stopped, only to see grandma return to life and ask where she is.

On top of these drugs, 24 percent of people over age 65 use gastro-intestinal drugs for things like ulcers, colitis, or constipation. Often the ulcer or the constipation is caused by medications being given for some other problem.

Many doctors just don't pay enough attention to drug interactions. They go on happily prescribing more drugs for what they see as more illnesses. The circle is complete; the patient is trapped. A perfect example was a patient of mine who was prescribed Stelazine, a tranquilizer, for extreme nervousness. After a few weeks on the medication, she went back to the doctor and told him that she felt even more tense and now had a feeling of "rigidity." The doctor, thinking that she was simply showing more of her neurotic nature, doubled the dose.

But her increasing symptoms were from the medication. She was having a condition called "tardive dyskinesia" that typically causes spasms of the neck and facial muscles. Doubling the dose put her into serious spasms, a state of terror, and could have led to permanent disability. She did not go back to the prescribing doctor for another doubling of the dose, but came to our office and was treated with an immediate intravenous dose of Benadryl. This cleared her symptoms in about 15 minutes. (There *is* a place for some drugs — often in emergencies — to counteract the bad effect of *other* drugs.)

What You Can Do

First, be aware of the myriad side-effects drugs can have. All too often a drug is prescribed, a side-effect occurs, the patient returns to the doctor and he promptly diagnoses the side-effect as another illness. The patient is given another drug and the cycle of pill — side-effect — pill continues until, in many cases, the side-effects become the real illness. Liver damage caused by prescription drugs, for instance, is not as rare as you might think. And once that kind of damage occurs, often there's no going back.

Drug-induced side-effects can include the following symptoms:

depression	diarrhea
hallucinations	constipation
confusion	skin rash
delirium	fatigue
memory loss	headache
impaired thinking	numbness
dizziness	blurred vision
falling	joint pain
incontinence	fainting
parkinsonism	swelling of the hands and face
involuntary movements	

This is just a partial list. So before you decide that someone you love is getting old, slow, and senile, you'd better check the medicine cabinet.

Finally, here's an exercise that might just surprise you. Get pencil and paper and take an inventory of the drugs you or your family members have used in the past six months. I mean prescription *and* over-the-counter drugs. Next, list the medical condition each drug is supposed to help.

Then, read this report and a few issues of my monthly newsletter to see which drugs are useless, unnecessary, overused, or harmful. You may be in for a surprise.

Hospital Errors

Drugs from the doctor or from the pharmacy can be dangerous but there's a place where drugs are even more likely to do you in — the hospital. This a place where you have absolutely no control over the drugs given to you. You can't ask the doctor or pharmacist what the prescription says or what the drug does because there is no prescription to look at. You are handed pills in a little cup by a nurse's aide who knows only slightly more about drugs than you do. The medication nurse has selected various drugs according to your doctor's orders and the aide has been instructed to give them to you and watch you take them. (So you can't get away with *not* taking them unless you are very clever.)

Recommendation: If you have been getting a routine set of pills, and suddenly you are given some that look different, *don't take them*. Either the doctor has changed your medication, which he isn't likely to do without telling you, or *you are getting some other patient's medicine.* That, of course, could be very serious.

Injections in the hospital are even more dangerous. There are many very lethal drugs in the medicine cabinet and a disastrous mistake may be only a hangover away. I saw a newborn baby die from a lethal injection of digitalis (Lanoxin) because the nurse moved the decimal point over one place and gave the baby ten times the prescribed dose. This is not an uncommon occurrence.

There are 500 or more medication-error deaths every year. This is four times the yearly average number of deaths on scheduled airlines. The number of medication errors made each year is in the tens of thousands, but no one knows the exact number because most of them are not reported and medication procedures are not carefully monitored. With tight budgets and the acute shortage of nurses, the situation is bound to get worse. Even though New York is better than most states in reporting and monitoring medication errors, a report in the *New England Journal of Medicine* revealed that the number of errors is probably *nine times* that reported. So in your state the situation may be even more serious.

Chapter 7
High Blood Pressure

Next to the common cold, high blood pressure is the most over-treated disease in America.

First, there isn't any real agreement on what constitutes high blood pressure. Is 140/90 high? Many, many physicians in this country would offer drugs for 140/90. But conservative physicians know that 140/90 is not high — especially for those over 50 years of age. Some doctors will use very powerful drugs to treat this "disease" even though the patient is experiencing no symptoms. But the patient will almost certainly have symptoms as a result of the drug, most commonly impotence, fatigue and other side effects that we will enumerate later.

A gentleman from Oklahoma wrote to me with the following question: "How can my wife lower her blood pressure? She has been on medication for years and is no better."

If I knew the answer to this question, the drug companies would not be making billions on blood pressure-lowering drugs. But here are some observations:

Blood pressure drugs sometimes work temporarily but the effectiveness tends to wear off as the placebo effect dissipates. Often they don't work at all. Note the comment: "She has been on medication for years and is no better." The very day I read this letter, I had a patient in my office who had been on two medications for his blood pressure, Lopressor and Indural, and yet his pressure was 190/100. I asked him what his pressure had been running since he had been placed on the drugs and he said: "About 170/70." When I informed him of his current pressure, he replied: "Well, yes, the doctor told me that it wasn't working but he's afraid to take me off the medication."

This would indicate to me that the doctor thinks the drugs have some magical properties other than what they are supposed to do, i.e., lower the blood pressure. Or, he may have the old Fear of Frying — in a courtroom. After all, it's okay to die on drugs, but it's not okay to die without them. The doctor *was* trying and the medications *are* the accepted treatment, backed by the great weight of scientific opinion. If he took you off the drugs and *then* you died, your death would be due to the doctor taking you off the drugs. Who is going to defend him in court for "doing nothing"? That is simply not acceptable to modern medicine, even if the medicine you are taking is making you miserable. In court, the "do nothing" doctor will be hung out to dry.

It is true that prolonged high blood pressure is "associated" with a higher death rate as compared to people with a normal pressure. But we don't know that the elevated pressure *causes* an earlier death. The elevated pressure simply might be a *protective* response to something else that we don't understand or even suspect.

If I had high blood pressure, I wouldn't take drugs. Although high blood pressure is associated with a higher death rate, *taking the drugs is also associated with a higher death rate.*

But whatever you do, don't stop the drugs abruptly. Sudden cessation of blood pressure medication can cause sudden death. I am amazed at how many patients come into my office who have not been warned of this danger.

What sort of side effects can you expect if you're taking these drugs? Depression for one (5 percent of patients); impotence for another; dizziness for a third (10 percent of patients); and just feeling lousy, which is the worst symptom of all, for yet another.

Blood pressure-lowering drugs can also cause tiredness, mental confusion, memory loss, headache, nightmares, and insomnia. Shortness of breath and bradycardia (a slowing of the heart rate) have been reported in three percent of patients. One percent of patients experience cold extremities, palpitations, congestive heart failure, swelling of the ankles, or *low* blood pressure. (Which can be far more dangerous than high blood pressure.)

You can also experience diarrhea, dry mouth, constipation, heart burn, and — worst of all possible complications — your hair may fall out.

The *Physicians' Desk Reference* gives the following helpful suggestion when prescribing blood pressure-lowering medications: "Discontinuation of the drug should be considered if any such reaction is not otherwise explicable." Thanks; I wouldn't have thought of that. But seriously, many doctors *don't* think of it.

What most patients don't realize is that the lowering of the blood by the drug is actually a side effect, just like the undesirable ones that you experience from the drug. The doctor just hopes that the "desirable" side effect of lowered blood pressure will exceed the undesirable side effects to a degree that you will continue on the drug. You should always keep that in mind when taking a drug: *The "therapeutic" effect is nothing but one of many side effects of the drug.* Hopefully, it is the dominant side effect and will work in your favor. Remember that the side effect of lowering the blood pressure can go too far and give you *too low* a blood pressure. If this effect is extreme, *you may have a stroke.*

There is an important point I alluded to above which needs to be discussed, but seldom is. At least, I've never heard any doctors talk about it. If the blood pressure is elevated, and no clear-cut reason is found for it (and there rarely is), isn't it possible that the elevated pressure is the body's method of compensating for something else? If this were the case, then wouldn't artificially lowering the pressure be exactly the wrong thing to do? Might this not explain why people on blood pressure medication often die, from whatever cause, sooner than those who left their pressure alone?

A 1982 study in the journal *Acta Medica Scandinavia* found that many patients over 50 were taking these drugs unnecessarily. It was found, in fact, that when the drugs were discontinued, 41 percent of the patients had their blood pressure return to normal within 11 months. This finding is a serious indictment of modern drug therapy, signifying a terrible waste of money and lives.

If your blood pressure is below 175/100, I think you are better off without medication. In fact I'm not convinced that medication for a pressure *over* that reading is going to do you any good unless you have symptoms proven to be related to the pressure. If the doctor finds physical evidence that the elevated pressure is doing you harm, such as damage to your heart or eyes, then maybe, and only maybe, the medication is warranted. You will be told that the drug is being given to you to *prevent* these unpleasant things from happening. But there is no proof that they actually work to prevent cardiovascular disease.

There are natural ways to lower your pressure. Nothing is 100 percent effective, but they won't do you any harm and they very often do work. Drink a lot of good mineral water, such as Lithia Springs water from Lithia Springs, Georgia. (No, I don't have any financial interest in the company— except that it gives me free water.) Use sea salt on your food. Keep your sugar intake low. Eat natural food, not overcooked. Get plenty of sunshine *without* sun shades. (Ignore the propaganda about killer ultraviolet light.) Exercise by walking, walking, walking—and loosen up.

If you have a concurrent disease with your elevated pressure, such as asthma, emphysema, chronic bronchitis, allergies, or congestive heart failure, you must be all the more cautious in taking blood pressure medication. These conditions can be made much worse and can kill you. The death would then be blamed on the condition and not the drug. Happens all the time.

Fortunately, high blood pressure doesn't usually cause any symptoms. It may surprise you to hear that before people became so doctor-conscious, and started getting "annual checkups" (a waste of time, often leading to unnecessary treatment and testing), they would go through a lifetime with "elevated" blood pressure and never know it. We don't know that their lives were shortened—and I doubt that they were.

A typical example of the Russian roulette you're playing when you take the latest drug offering is the Bristol lab product, Enkaid. The package insert for this anti- heart flutter product says that "an excessive mortality ... was seen in patients treated with Enkaid compared with that seen in a carefully matched placebo-treated group."

This statement is at the same time horrifying and amusing. Forty out of 415 patients taking the drug died — *almost 10 percent.* Yet the drug was left on the market for five months after the above report was made. On September 16, 1991, Bristol Laboratories announced that they were taking Enkaid off the market. You could get a refund on the unused portion of your prescription — if you were still alive!

There's a certain amount of graveside humor there, but the placebo part really cracked me up. They matched the drug with a placebo and came up with the conclusion that Enkaid killed more than the placebo. We told you placebo studies were futile and asinine — how many patients did they think the placebo, a starch pill, was going to kill?

Bristol's lack of concern for human life is not an isolated event by any means. Hoffman-La Roche, one of the world's largest drug companies, continued to sell a sedative in the U.S., even though they knew it had killed people in Europe. The drug, called Versed, was marketed in a strength *five times* what it should have been. Even though this was known, and an internal Roche memo stated that the drug had caused "oversedation, prolonged apnea (cessation of breathing), *and death"* the FDA approved the drug at the deadly 5X strength. Then the death reports began to come in.

I don't think you have to be "a conspiracy theorist with a lively imagination" to call this incompetence, malfeasance, and worse. I call it murder.

Beta-Blockers

If your doctor has placed you on beta-blockers, you've got more trouble. These drugs supposedly treat hard-to-correct cases of high blood pressure. They're dangerous — especially for those of you over 50.

If you have asthma, emphysema, chronic bronchitis, allergies, or congestive heart disease you're in even greater danger from beta-blockers. If you smoke, things are worse yet. Beta-blockers can alter your thinking — and I don't mean they make you smarter. Depression, hallucinations, insomnia, and nightmares are just a few of the changes you may see.

Beta-blockers can cause spasms in the air passages of your lungs. That makes it hard to breathe. Even worse, beta-blockers can cause liver and kidney damage.

So, what's the upside of beta-blockers? They work on some of the people some of the time but not on all of the people all of the time. The bottom line is to avoid all blood pressure medications if you possibly can.

A partial list of medications for blood pressure is as follows:

Aldactazide	Hytrin	Renese
Aldoril	Inderide	Salutensin
Apresazide	Isoptin	Ser-Ap-Es
Capotin	Lozol	Serpasil
Capozide	Minipres	Tenex
Catapres	Minizide	Tenoretic
Combipres	Hydromox	Timolide
Corzide	Monopril	Trandate
Diupres	Normodyne	Vasotec
Dyazide	Normozide	Vaseretic
DynaCirc	Oreticyl	Wytensin
Enduronyl	Prinvil	Yocon
Esidrix	Prinzide	Zestoretic
Esimil	Rauzide	Zestril
Hydropres		

And last, but not least, Digitalis (also known as Digoxin and Lanoxin).

This heart rhythm-suppressing drug is one of the most widely prescribed drugs in the world, and for good reason — it works. Drugs come and go, but Digitalis is the tenth most commonly prescribed drug year after year. It has proven its effectiveness in over 200 years of service.

So what's the problem? Well, it's *not* needed in about half of the cases where used, and it's a dangerous drug. The main reason it's dangerous is that doctors will often put a patient on *"dij"* and forget about it. If the patient isn't monitored properly, the dij level may gradually increase until toxic levels are reached. *This can be fatal.*

A recent article in the *Journal of the American Medical Association* reviewed cardiac arrests in a major teaching hospital in Boston for the year 1981. Fourteen percent of these disastrous events were caused by, paradoxically, the very drugs that are supposed' to prevent such a catastrophe — including Lanoxin.

While on the subject of rhythm-controlling drugs, I want to tell you about a drug trial that shows what a minefield this group of heart medications represents. A $45 million trial was done on the drugs Tambocor and Enkaid. The researchers hypothesized that there would be a 30 percent reduction in mortality among the lucky recipients of either of these wonder drugs for abnormal heartbeats. The trial had to be halted when the mortality increased by 200 percent. Aren't you glad you didn't participate? By the way: Don't *ever* participate in a drug trial.

We were taught in medical school (and it's still being taught) that once a patient was put on Digitalis, he would have to stay on it for life. The idea was, if you need it, you need it, and nothing can change that. Like so many other things we learned in medical school, that simply wasn't true.

Chapter 8
Tranquilizers and Sleeping Pills

Welcome to "La-La Land." That's not a bad monicker for a country which uses tranquilizers, sedatives, and sleeping pills like they're candy.

Drug companies make billions of dollars from the likes of Valium (Prince Val), Halcion (Prince Hal), Stelazine (Princess Stella), Compazine (maybe you can think of a good royal title), Librium (the Liberator — from your problems), Tranxene (the medication transfer — to Dorksville), Xanex (X out your problems), Mellaril (Prince Mel), Thorazine (the mighty god, Thor), Loxitane (take lox of it and make Lederle rich) and sinequan (the sine qua non for quashing your gilt about killing your mother while on Halcion — a good hit of doxepin hydrochloride will turn the trick). I'll bet you thought these names had some scientific meaning. No, they're just the creation of some Madison Avenue type with a distorted sense of humor.

The number of prescriptions written for the tranquilizer Halcion are in the millions. Before Halcion, Valium was the most prescribed drug in America. But Prince Val lost out to Prince Hal. Hal, they said, didn't cause hangovers like that nasty Prince Val. And as it turned out, Val was also very addicting. The coup was quick and decisive — Val was out and Hal was in. At least they came from the same family — the benzodiazepine dynasty. Hal performed beyond belief for one so young — seven million prescriptions in 1990 alone.

Even former Secretary of State, James Baker, popped Halcion when flying on a trip. (And when wasn't he on a trip? I always wondered what he was on.) Consider the absurdity of it: Our Secretary of State is out there dealing with a bunch of fanatics in the Middle East (and I'm talking about *both* sides — I don't want the Salmon Rushdie treatment) in which he is establishing the ground rules for World War III, and while on this sensitive mission he is popping Halcion for sleep. So he is subject to, *according to Upjohn's own package insert,* "bizarre or abnormal behavior, agitation, hallucinations, amnesia of upcoming events, called antegrade amnesia, *reported by individuals who have been taking Halcion to induce sleep while traveling) such as during an airplane flight"* (Emphasis added.) As boring as Baker is, maybe he needs a little Halcion-induced agitation, but "bizarre and abnormal behavior" isn't likely to produce world peace.

Drug promoters are really clever. Halcyon, with a "Y" instead of an "I," means a period of peace and tranquility, as in "halcyon days." Valium is valiant, Stelazine is stellar, Equanil is equitable — you get the picture.

But a serious tremor was recently felt beneath the throne —-about a 6.57 on the Richter scale, emanating from the Rocky Mountains of Utah. A Utah woman took Halcion — and then killed her mother. (A few paragraphs ago, you thought I was just kidding — or had "a lively imagination.")

Halcion's halcyon days were over. The Upjohn company quickly shored up the dam by settling out of court and denying that Hal had anything to do with the murder (women kill their mothers all the time).

Then came the Richter 8.7. The British Department of Health announced that they would suspend the use of Halcion in Great Britain, citing new evidence that Halcion "is associated with a much higher frequency of side effects, particularly memory loss and depression." And, they said, "1/2 mg of triazolam [Hal's real name] produced *very robust and highly reliable memory impairments* [don't British adjectives crack you up?] — a reduction of 63 percent in recall." (Baker to Bush: "Yes, Mr. President, that's my signature alright, but I don't remember giving away Turkey, Albania, and Mississippi.")

Another British report stated that "of 390 adverse reactions reported ... 41 percent were psychiatric." Hmmm, psychiatric. There's another one of those British adjectives. Let me see if I can put that in laymen's terms: boffers, bonko, beanie, and brain-baked — not the kind of person you would want baby-sitting your kids (or your country). Being a little psycho isn't as bad as actual murder, but the Brits had seen enough; they banned Halcion. Hal lost a *whole nation* — wham, just like that. Then, more bad news: Finland and Norway booted Hal out; Canada and Germany will soon follow suit.

Meanwhile back in the colonies, Hal was facing rebellion. (But, of course, not from psychiatrists, who think Halcion is just great. How could anyone consider banning such a drug simply because it causes what we are supposed to be trying to cure?)

Prince Hal had adjusted his crown and bravely held his head high following the British report — only to be whacked alongside it again by an American professor of medicine from Pennsylvania State University — a cruel blow indeed. Dr. Anthony Kales reported, "No other benzodiazepine has such a narrow margin of safety. The only justification for keeping it on the market is to insure the company's profitability. From a public health standpoint, there is no reason at all. It's clear that this is a dangerous drug."

Looking back at the approval history of Hal reveals a shocking disregard for the opinions of the FDA's *own experts* on the issue of safety of the product. Ten years ago, Dr. Theresa Woo, the medical review officer for Halcion, recommended non-approval but was overruled by her superiors. If she was the medical review officer, then presumably she was the person in the agency who knew the most about the drug. What did she know that we haven't been told? How many people have suffered damage or death because she was not listened to? Who got paid what for going against her advice? It wouldn't be the first time FDA officials have been caught with their hands in drug company pockets — remember the generic drug company bribe scandal? (Maybe Halcion will land some more FDA medicrats in jail.)

Upjohn now admits submitting "incomplete data" on Halcion's side effects. Was Dr. Woo the only intelligent (and honest) doctor to notice that? A company spokesman in England says the incomplete data was a "transcription error."

That's the sort of hanky panky that leads to tragedies like the British Thalidomide babies.

Do these companies have any social conscience at all? Upjohn has resisted any changes in the warning label for fear of hurting sales and, rather than face up to unflattering research, they have attacked it. Before the murder trial mentioned above, Upjohn tried to use the copyright laws to suppress damaging documents, even though they admitted they contained no trade secrets. These drug companies are ruthless.

The head of the FDA, Dr. David A. Kessler, also has a certificate in business administration from New York University. Is he practicing good medicine in his job or just good business? Why is Halcion still on the market when it has been banned in three Western countries?

It is said that Halcion only causes people to turn nasty when the patient takes more than he is supposed to, has been drinking alcohol, or has been on it for a long time. How are you going to control neurotic patients so they won't take more at a time than the doc said to take? How are you going to control a neurotic patient's alcohol intake? If the patient has been on the drug "for a long time" ... well, what can I tell you?

Upjohn's promotion of Halcion turned out to be prophetic, at least in once sense. Referring to their claim that Halcion didn't interfere with "daytime alertness," they said, in a beautiful full-color ad in the *New England Journal of Medicine*; "Improved sleep is only half the Halcion story." They sure got *that* right. (All this phoney hucksterism doesn't make the *New England Journal of Medicine* look very good either. I *told* them not to let themselves be seduced by the drug industry.)

It's amusing to watch the happy-pill giants go after each other right in the medical journals. The Upjohn company attacks Librium, Dalmane and Valium in a two-page ad in which they point out that these three drugs cause a dramatic increase in hip fractures because of their long sedating effect. One study found a dramatic 80 percent increase in fractures as compared with patients not taking one of these products. But Upjohn produces Halcion and you know what *that* does.

Who is the heir-apparent to Prince Hal? It has to be *somebody*. We aren't going to stop taking funny pills. Just because Americans did without them for 175 years and didn't kill their mothers over which TV channel to watch doesn't mean we are going to give up something that will make reality seem like never-never land.

The new feel-good prince will be Xanax, the one that X's away your worry about the car payment. Who wants to face one of *those* every month without a little help?

Will Xanax be any safer than Halcion? According to Upjohn's (yep, same company) own literature, Xanax can cause a confusional state, memory impairment, "cognitive disorder," abnormal involuntary movements, "disinhibition" and agitation — sound like anybody we know? An FDA analysis in 1990 found that Halcion was responsible for more hostile acts by patients than any other drug. Guess what was number two — I'll give you a hint. It's initials were "Xanax."

Now, of course, your family doctor is a bit more reticent about prescribing Valium-type drugs. But his newfound concern is typical of a drug-oriented medical philosophy. Year after year these harmful drugs are gladly given by physicians. Then, after some consumer group or TV shows like "20/20" expose the problem, physicians suddenly turn caring. What about those patients who took the pills and became psychotic? How about families that were destroyed because unsuspecting mothers became addicted to Valium and turned from loving moms to paranoid pill-poppers?

We don't really know how much crime, divorce, and suicide is caused by these powerful drugs because *nobody has been keeping score.* So many millions of people are on these chemical agents, including people on welfare who are *expected* to commit violent crimes, that no one has any idea how much homicide is a result of the pills (especially when those pills are combined with alcohol).

I can assure you that Roche, the peddlers of Valium and Librium, aren't going to be asking for an investigation of this problem. They can't resist making obscene profits, regardless of their products' effects on an unsuspecting public.

Roche's marketing campaign looked like it was designed by General George Patton. Roche sent doctors brochures which stated that Valium was "an important component for treatment programs for the relief of excessive geriatric anxiety and psychic tension." Worried about getting old? Have a pill! And what's psychic tension? I've been in medicine for 30 years and I don't know what psychic tension is, and neither do the ad boys at Roche. I can't believe that doctors fall for this swamp gas.

Later the company would hold "Roche Seminars on Aging." These "informative" get-togethers were ways to convince doctors that Valium was an essential part of treatment for older Americans, like treating a vitamin deficiency.

Why the sudden interest in the elderly? Was Roche concerned about these people? Maybe so. Drug manufacturers have moms and dads like everybody else. But being a concerned cynic, I can't help but think there might be a different reason.

Demographic studies in the early 1980s clearly showed that the number of older Americans was growing. Roche saw an opportunity to market their space pills to a new group of consumers. Like magic, Valium became the miracle drug for the over-60 set. Did it work? Like a hot knife through butter. Between 1980 and 1985, the number of people over age 60 using tranquilizers skyrocketed — especially among older women.

Warning: If you are taking Valium, Dalmane, or any other of the benzodiazepines, and are also on digoxin, the Valium-type drug can cause you to have a digoxin overdose.

You might be wondering, "If these pills are being used by millions of Americans, certainly they must be helping someone." Unfortunately, these pills do little good for anyone. A recent study which considered alternatives to tranquilizers found that patients suffering from anxiety, who were given advice and reassurance by their doctors, *were calmed just as well as those given tranquilizers.*

Another study divided patients into four groups — three were given tranquilizers, the fourth received a placebo. The results showed that the placebo — the sugar pill — worked as well as the tranquilizers. Anxiety in most people comes and goes on its own; no drugs are needed. Time heals all wounds, even psychic ones, but the doctor and his uppers and downers get the credit.

It's like backaches — 80 percent of them go away with or without treatment. But the chiropractor, the physical therapist, or the "orthopedist gets the credit, and an 80 percent cure rate looks good in any specialty.

Believe me, sleeping pills are no better than tranquilizers. In fact some of them *are* tranquilizers. There is one called Dalmane that is nothing but a slight variation from Valium. How did it become a sedative instead of a tranquilizer? Phony research and marketing creates financial winners.

Most people have times when falling asleep is difficult. These periods rarely last; they almost always go away of their own volition. In older people, falling asleep at night is often difficult because many older folks take naps during the day. Naturally, if you're prone to taking catnaps, you're going to have difficulty sleeping at night. The solution: don't sleep during the day. (Not that there's anything wrong with a nap during the day. You just can't sleep during the day and during the night, too — with a few notable exceptions; some people can sleep at a Grateful Dead concert.)

Prozac

There have been a number of cases of purported suicide and murder blamed on the "anxiolytic" drug, Prozac. The situation has gotten so tense, and the manufacturer, Eli Lilly, has gotten so anxious, that I imagine Lilly's execs are thinking about taking some of their own medicine.

In response, the company has taken an unprecedented step: It announced that it will pay all legal costs for doctors sued for prescribing the drug. That shows a lot of confidence — and some very deep pockets.

But think about it for a minute. A lot of doctors must be getting sued for Lilly to make such an offer. Yet its choice to pay legal costs rather than pull the drug means marketing the drug must be profitable, even in the face of numerous, presumably very expensive, lawsuits. Like I said, this is not a penny-ante game — nor is it a place for altruists.

The FDA, naturally, backs the company and says there is no relation between Prozac use and suicide or crime. Maybe they are right; time will tell — maybe 10 or 20 years.

The major brand names of tranquilizers, anxiolytics, mood elevators and sleepers are those listed below:

Atarax	Librium	Prozac
Ativan	Limbitrol	Raudixin
Benadryl	Loxitane	Serax
Butisol	Mebaral	Serentil
Centrax	Mellaril	Sinequan
Compazine	Miltown	Stelazine
Dalmane	Moban	Thorazine
Deprol	Navane	Trancopal
Doriden	Noludar	Tranxene
Equanil	Prozac	Triavil
Eskalith	Pamelor	Trilafon
Etrafon	Phenergan	Valium
Halcion	Placidy	Vistaril
Haldol	Prolixin	Xanax
Innovar		

Serious Side Effects

You are probably familiar with most of the side effects of tranquilizers, sedatives, and so-called mood elevators. These range from addiction, confusion, memory loss, and dizziness to slurred speech, slowed learning, and depression. But such drugs can also cause drug-induced senility. And finally, if you mix a bit of alcohol with these pills, you can get the side-effect of all side-effects — sudden death is not at all uncommon.

For older Americans, drug-induced senility is the most subversive side-effect. As we age, we expect to get mentally slower. So, when we take these tranquilizers and find our minds are not as quick as they used to be, we think it's normal. But it's often a side effect of the drug given to make the elderly patient "happy." Drug-induced senility is a by-product of the spreading tranquilizer use in this country. Older Americans are not necessarily mentally slower; they don't fall more frequently than younger folks unless they have weakness or a physical handicap. But when you are drugged day in and day out, the result can only be mental and physical confusion — and a broken hip.

What about addiction? The myth is that those who are addicted to tranquilizers are prone to addictive behavior. If it isn't Valium, it will be alcohol, tobacco, or street drugs. This is true of many people but certainly not of everybody.

This myth, in fact, was perpetuated by the makers of Valium, in an attempt to "prove" that their drug was not addictive to most Americans. In 1979, the then-president of Hoffman-La Roche testified before the Senate hearing on abuse of tranquilizers. This man, Robert Clark, had the nerve to tell Senators that "true addiction is probably exceedingly unusual and, when it occurs, is probably confined to those individuals with abuse-prone personalities who ingest large amounts."

The truth is that the *majority* of people who use drugs like Valium for more than two months will start to become addicted. Again, to quote the consumer group Public Citizen, "the majority of the 2 million older adults in this country who regularly use these pills have become addicted ... thanks to their doctors and the drug industry."

What's the bottom line with tranquilizers and sleeping pills? Even the FDA says, "Anxiety or tension associated with the stress of everyday life usually does not require treatment with a [tranquilizer]." So what if it took the bureaucrats at FDA 20 years to figure it out? At least they're ahead of the drug industry.

Take a look at this partial list of possible tranquilizers. Which of them are preferable in normal anxiety or tension?

suicidal thoughts	homicidal thoughts	depression
sedation	dizziness	weakness
addiction	unsteadiness	disorientation
nausea	loss of appetite	headache
insomnia	agitation	skin rash
double vision	blurring of vision	heart burn
flushing	constipation	hypotension
amnesia	tardive dyskinesia**	seizures
anxiety	fever	muscle rigidity
tachycardia*	hypertension	liver disease
low blood count	acne	hair loss
photosensitivity	impotence	hyperglycemia
hypoglycemia	diarrhea	urine retention
bronchial spasm	sudden death***	cataracts
confusion	speech difficulty	incontinence
jaundice	slurred speech	tremor
hyperexcitation	hallucinations	rage

  * A rapid heart beat. Other types of cardiac abnormalities may be seen on the electrocardiogram.

 ** A grotesque writhing and spasm of the muscles of the face causing the patient to appear to be an imbecile. Once established, there is no known treatment. Muscles in other parts of the body may also be involved.

*** Especially with Haldol.

SPECIAL NOTICE: If you know someone who is over 60 years old who has developed hallucinations, delirium, or other schizophrenic-like behavior, there is a very, very good chance that these symptoms are being caused by prescription drugs — particularly tranquilizers and sedatives — or the withdrawal from addiction to drugs like Valium, Indocin, Darvon, or Roxanal.

Depression

Depression is another psychological buzzword. What is depression? What constitutes severe depression? When should drugs be used to treat depression? Answers? We don't know. There is no commonly agreed upon definition of depression; one doctor's diagnosis of severe depression is another's normal reaction to life's problems.

When should drugs be used? Almost never — and only in the most severe, long-term cases. These patients are the ones most likely to commit suicide with the very drug the doctor has given them for their "problem." (I suppose the doctors and the drug companies would argue that they cured the patients' depression.)

Most people who are sad and/or depressed do not need therapy of any kind, unless that therapy is an understanding friend, family member, or minister — or a few minutes of exercise each day. The irony is that patients are often given drugs to treat depression which has been caused by other drugs. If someone you know has suddenly become depressed, don't run to the psychologist. Instead, run to the medicine cabinet and see which drugs he or she is taking. The odds are that's where the problem is.

Here's a partial list of drugs known to cause depression in some individuals:

All blood pressure medications
Valium, Halcion and all of the other tranquilizers
Inderal
Norpace
Zantac
Tagamet
Dopar
Amphetamines
Steroids like prednisone
Many antibiotics
Ibuprofen (Motrin, Nalfon, etc.)
Many over-the-counter products

Weight Reduction Pills

Many people become depressed because of a weight problem and are desperate to solve the problem. So they start taking weight reduction pills. The leader in this field is the heavily-advertised Dexatrim. It's a form of speed called phenylpropanolamine. It has *no place* in the treatment of weight loss and should be banned from sale. It causes headache, nervousness, a rapid heartbeat, dizziness, palpitations, insomnia, and, of course, loss of appetite. It also has a strong addiction potential. Becoming a speed freak is a high price to pay for a little *temporary* weight loss.

Chapter 9
Arthritis

Let's start at the top: *There is no cure for rheumatoid arthritis.* I hate to sound negative, but that's a simple fact. It's why many rheumatologists are out looking for an honest line of work.

Yes, you can reduce the swelling, but the best and cheapest way to do that is to take an aspirin. The slew of arthritis drugs in the market today are worse than useless — they're harmful and very expensive. And study after study shows that these "miracle" drugs are *no more effective than aspirin.* I'm not in love with aspirin; I think you know that. But if you need something to reduce the swelling of arthritis, aspirin is not a bad choice. And combined with some mild exercise and the proper diet, you might just feel pretty good.

Arthritis drugs, such as Feldene, can cost almost $1,000 a year per patient. Aspirin costs about $2 per hundred. You don't have to be an accountant to notice a slight difference in cost here.

And don't fall for that good-looking Tylenol lady either. She and Angela Lansbury are professional actors who, I guarantee you, know a lot less about drugs than the readers of this report.

What about steroids? *Avoid these drugs.* Steroids can, and often do, cause osteoporosis — the thinning of your bones. Steroids (cortisone), can also cause diabetes, hypertension, acne and other infections, cataracts, Cushings syndrome, sexual dysfunction, and psychosis.

Remember, there is no cure for arthritis. Don't be fooled by quacks — even if they are members of the AMA and are certified by the American Rheumatology Association.

There is an insane and totally irresponsible trend in arthritis therapy, born out of frustration and failure, to use anti-cancer (chemotherapy) drugs for the treatment of arthritis. These drugs are called DMARDs (pronounced: *dee-mards)*, which stands for Disease-Modifying Agents for Rheumatoid Disease.

The most popular DMARD is methotrexate (alias amethopterin), trade name: Rheumatrex. The contra-indications and side effects take up *two pages of small print* in the Physicians Desk Reference. It's so toxic that they have a special drug, called Leucovorin, designed to try to bring you back from the brink of death. It's called the "Leucovorin Rescue Schedule." Isn't *that* a comforting thought!

There is one little side effect that Leucovorin can't rescue you from; it's called cancer. Curing your arthritis with cancer seems like a bad tradeoff. That, according to investigators in Toronto, Canada, is exactly what you are doing if you take this drug. Their report indicated an increase in lung cancer and leukemia from taking DMARDs but, they added, *"denying this therapy is usually considered unethical"!* Don't ask me how they come to that conclusion.

As usual, there's a much simpler way to deal with the problem, and it doesn't include taking drugs (or getting cancer). Many studies have shown that fasting can dramatically improve arthritis. If you're desperate, quit eating; it works.

Cortisone-like Drugs

Non-steroidal anti-inflammatory drugs, called NSAIDs (pronounced *en-seds)* for short, have taken over a large portion of the arthritis market in the past few years. When Motrin (ibuprofen) was released by the FDA for over-the-counter sale, it quickly skyrocketed to the top of the drug sales charts. Motrin, and the other NSAIDs, were pronounced safe and effective by our "protectors" at the FDA. Now, a decade later, a different story is emerging. Gastritis and ulcer formation are two of the not-so-safe side effects of Motrin, Nalfon, Tolectin and the other NSAIDs that were going to be a panacea for arthritis.

But there is an even more serious side effect — these drugs can ruin your kidneys. Nephritis, renal necrosis (death of kidney tissue) and acute renal failure are being reported, especially in older men. Daily use of NSAIDs is associated with a twofold increase in risk for chronic renal disease. For some unexplained reason, this risk is limited to men.

These are some of the more commonly prescribed arthritis drugs:

Aspirin	Ecotrin	Motrin
Butazolidin	Empirin	Nalfon
Celestone	Feldene	Naprosin
Clinoril	Imuran	Pabalate
Cortisone	Indocin	Rheumatrex
DMSO	Kenalog	Tolectin
Decadron	Meclomin	Trilisate
Dolobid	Medrol	

Chapter 10
Cancer Chemotherapy Drugs

We mentioned above that the cancer drug, methotrexate, is now being used for arthritis and that it will induce cancer in some of these unlucky patients. I am not going to take a lot of space telling you how deadly and ineffective the cancer drugs are. It's hard to imagine any educated and reasonably well-read person not knowing at least some of the abysmal truth about these drugs.

But a recent British report is worth mentioning because it reveals that they are even more deadly than we could have possibly imagined. Medical personnel handling these cancer drugs are more likely to contract leukemia or lymphoma (lymph node cancer) than personnel not exposed to them. The period from exposure to cancer varies from seven to 33 years. If simply handling these drugs will induce cancer, how can they be expected to cure cancer — more of a bad thing? Fire with fire? It's too scientific for me.

Here's some more high science. A patient consent form for the use of the cancer drug, interleukin-2, reads: "It is very unlikely, though possible, that this treatment could cause your death. In previous studies, these side effects have been transient and have returned to normal after discontinuation of interleukin-2." Hmmm, well, as long as death is only transient....

I received a sad letter from a gentleman wanting to know if I could help his mother who was dying of cancer of the breast. He described in considerable detail all of the surgeries, radiation therapy and chemicals that his mother had received. My reply pretty much sums up my feeling toward cancer chemotherapy:

Dear Mr. H:

Thanks for your letter concerning your mother. You asked for a second opinion and so here it is:

Your mother has received absolutely atrocious treatment in the grand manner of modern science. She would live longer if they left her alone. Dr. George Crile of the Cleveland Clinic proved this in the case of breast cancer many years ago. Her "second look" surgery, when they knew the case was hopeless, was an unforgivable assault on your mother.

As for the "chemotherapy," using your mother in a 'double blind' study of a toxic chemical is no different than using mice or dogs for experimentation, except your mother is a beloved human being and should not be treated in such a callous manner. I am sorry to be so blunt, Mr. H, but I get very angry when I hear such stories of gross maltreatment in supposedly good medical centers such as Johns Hopkins University. You have probably been wiped out financially and, not having anything to offer your mother, I don't want to add to your burden.

Loss of a parent is never easy. I wish you the best during this difficult and depressing ordeal.

You might think I was a little extreme in this letter but my opinion is backed by sound clinical studies which confirm the gross quackery going on in the treatment of cancer today. The University of Kansas Medical Center released a report to the *Journal of the American Geriatrics Society* in which it stated "the prognosis for these [cancer] patients has changed very little since the 1940s...." In case your arithmetic is a little rusty, that's 50 years of no progress. They also said that the drugs caused "immediate morbidity and shortened life in the majority of these elderly patients."

How can these Doctors of Death get away with this? One reason is because everyone, including other doctors, assume that valid studies have been done proving the efficacy of "chemotherapy" drugs.

Let me illustrate why this is impossible to do. There are about 30 chemicals now being used in cancer therapy. They were initially tested on "soft" tumors, or sarcomas. These tumors will often be ameliorated, but not cured, by a drug. The major killer, "hard" tumors such as cancer of the lung, stomach, ovary, breast, and prostate, are not cured, or even inhibited, by these drugs.

It is now fashionable to use three drugs in the treatment of cancer. If you select three out of the 30 drugs available for cancer treatment, the three will have to be tested against all the others to determine which will be the most effective for the case being treated. This process involves 24,360 possible combinations. Now if the order of giving the drugs is important, and the chemotherapists say that it is, then you have six separate permutations to consider along with the 24,360 combinations of three drugs. Now you have 146,160 different ways to give three drugs to a patient. This is why it is impossible to know anything about the effectiveness of any chemotherapy treatment.

Chapter 11

Antibiotics

Perhaps more than any other class of drugs, antibiotics are dangerously over-prescribed or misprescribed. In congressional hearings related to the misuse of prescription drugs, it was determined that between 40-60 percent of all antibiotics were improperly prescribed — that is, prescribed for infections which cannot effectively be treated by antibiotics. That bears repeating: up to 60 percent of all antibiotics prescribed in this country are misprescribed. Doesn't say much for this country's medical education, does it?

And most people are so enamored with antibiotics they literally demand them from their doctors. Worse, most Americans have no idea about the large range of severe side effects antibiotics can, and often do, cause.

Lets start with stomach irritation and diarrhea. Not severe enough for you? Then think about those cases of stomach irritation that progress into severe intestinal problems caused by bacteria that is almost impossible to kill. Almost any type of antibiotic can cause an inflammation of the colon known as antibiotic- associated colitis.

Then there's severe liver and kidney damage, particularly in older patients.

How about irreversible bone marrow depression — a side effect of the antibiotic chloramphenicol — which can be fatal. For a time they gave this "wonder drug" in the hospital knowing that in almost 50 percent of the cases it wasn't necessary! Now, after 20 years of misuse, prescribing this drug is considered malpractice in most instances.

Nearly 10 percent of the American population is allergic to various forms of penicillin. These allergic reactions can be irritating — like skin rashes, itching, and swelling; or they can be serious — like muscle pain, abdominal pain, shortness of breath, and death. And if you've experienced allergic reactions to penicillin, it's likely you will also be allergic to cephalosporins — a class of antibiotics related to penicillin.

In older adults, the dosage used is also critical. High doses of penicillins and/or cephalosporins can cause seizures, drowsiness, and confusion. And if you suffer from any type of kidney impairment, a normal dose of penicillin could cause hyperkalemia — a possibly fatal increase of potassium in your system.

One of the most hazardous byproducts of this ridiculous faith in the power of antibiotics has been the development of strains of bacteria that are antibiotic resistant. What do you do when you get a disease that antibiotics are helpless against?

In short, Americans use antibiotics for all the wrong reasons; doctors over-prescribe them, especially to children, and by the time we're adults we've taken so many antibiotics that they don't work anymore. The result is that when we finally need the help of antibiotics for illnesses that are truly life-threatening, they don't work.

This could, and probably does, explain why we are now seeing, after years of intensive battles against infectious diseases, a recrudescence of these same diseases (syphilis, staphylococcus, streptococcus, tuberculosis, lymphogranuloma, cholera, strep A, measles, diphtheria, mumps) and the emergence of heretofore unknown diseases, such as chlamydia, herpes II, Legionnaires' disease, Palestine syndrome, mycoplasmas, prions, HTLV-I and II, Crutzfeld-Jacob disease and many others. The extensive use of antibiotics are undoubtedly responsible for some of these discouraging phenomena, including some of the viral diseases mentioned above that don't respond to antibiotics, anyway.

The overuse and abuse of antibiotics in treating children is especially a cause for concern. In addition to being immune suppressant and yeast-stimulating, antibiotics may delay the disease to a later date when the child is older and less able to mount an effective immune response. Some scientists think that the organism is never destroyed by the antibiotic, but is instead driven into another form which hides and waits for another day. Antoine Beauchamp and others in the 19th Century felt that the effort to thwart disease processes would always lead to the substitution of another organism that would ravage the body as much as the suppressed organism — maybe more.

Immunizations (which are drugs of a biological nature) are also seriously implicated in this new age of pestilence. I won't go into a great deal of detail in this report, but you can read more on immunizations and their questionable value in my special report, *Lethal Injections.*

But I can't resist reporting one vaccine fiasco to you. There was an outbreak of influenza A at a nursing home in Maryland. Of the 126 patients who caught the flu, 72 percent had been vaccinated. There was no significant difference in the influenza attack rate between vaccinated and unvaccinated patients.

But something else was very significant. I have pointed out that if a person contracts the disease for which he was vaccinated, the disease is likely to be more severe and can be fatal. In this nursing home epidemic, five of the patients developed pneumonia. Four out of the five had been vaccinated, and two of those four died. None of the unvaccinated patients died.

Antibiotics, like so many things in medicine (and life), are a two-edged sword. There is no doubt that they have saved millions of lives in the past 50 years. As I mentioned above, if you get bacterial meningitis, and you don't get penicillin in time, you are going to die. But the antibiotic sword also cuts the other way. If you don't need antibiotics, but get them anyway, you could be much the worse for the experience; you could even die. The key is to use informed judgement as to when their use is indicated. *That* is something our medical community shows little inclination to do.

Chapter 12

Asthma

Asthma is making a dramatic comeback. The incidence of asthma has risen by an astounding six percent a year since the early 1970s, resulting in a dramatic increase in the use of anti-asthma drugs.

With all the new and frightening diseases we have to cope with, asthma has been overlooked as a serious and life-threatening disease. But asthma hasn't liked being ignored and the number of fatalities from this terrible and debilitating disease (ask someone who has it) have increased dramatically. We are definitely losing ground. The medications are not working — and they have become part of the problem.

Beta-2 drugs, such as Alupent, Brethaire, and Brethine, work remarkably well in relieving an asthmatic attack, but are they killing the patients? They act by opening up the air passages, similar to the action of adrenaline, but, according to some doctors, the patients may be paying for this relief with their lives.

A Canadian study, which was actually financed by a drug company, revealed an appalling fact: Asthmatic patients who used two Beta-2 inhalers a month *faced a risk of death double that of patients who used only one inhaler a month.*

Clive Page of King's College, London, has been warning for five years that the Beta-2 drugs may be killing asthmatics. He says the drugs hasten the process by which asthma kills. As with cortisone, and its dramatic effect on many diseases, the immediate relief given to asthmatic patients by these drugs may not be worth the price. In fact, I'll guarantee you it isn't worth the price when that price is *death.*

Another of these drugs, Fenoteral, was studied in New Zealand. Researchers found that six months of treatment made the patient *worse* than patients taking a placebo.

Following are some of the most commonly used asthma drugs:

AeroBid	Choledyl	Pro vent il
Alupent	Decadron	Slo-bid
Aminophyllin	Dilor	Sus-Phrine
Beclovent	Elixophyllin	T-Phyl
Brethaire	Intal	Theo-24
Brethine	Isuprel	Tornalate
Bricanyl	Metaprel	Uniphyl
Bronkephrine	Norisodrine	Vanceril
Bronkometer	Primatene	Ventolin
Bronkosol		

Low Back Pain

Low back pain is one of the most common complaints in medicine, yet there is almost no agreement on how best to treat it. To exercise a sore back or not to exercise it is one of the areas in dispute. Six studies indicated that exercise was of value, but *ten* studies found *no* therapeutic benefit from exercise whatsoever. I know exercise isn't a drug, at least not for most of us, but so-called muscle relaxants *are* drugs and they are of even less value than exercise for back pain. I use the term "so-called" because many of them are only variants of Valium.

Just to put it all in perspective, studies have shown that over *80 percent of back pain will go away with out any treatment at all*. These are some of the most commonly used muscle relaxants:

Anectine	Paraflex	Skelaxin
Dantrium	Parafon	Soma
Flexeril	Quinamm	Tracrium
Lioresal	Robaxin	Valium
Metubine	Robaxisol	Valrelease

Conclusion

This report may have shocked you, but it is only part of the story. Another hundred pages could have been written about the cheating and coverups that take place all too often in the palaces (and many of them look like palaces) of the "ethical" drug companies.

And another hundred pages yet could have been devoted to the cheating that goes on at the "clinical investigator" level. Some of these doctors make as much as a million dollars a year. But if they come up with too many negative findings, such as excess toxicity or ineffectiveness of the drug, they will soon find themselves no longer on that company's drug investigation team. This is a clear conflict of interest, which leads to many of the tragedies we see with modern drugs, such as Thalidomide, Oraflex, Halcion, Selecrin and many others.

And the last hundred pages could have been devoted to the greed, arrogance, stupidity, and inefficiency of the Food and Drug Administration ... no, I guess that would take more like a thousand pages. Clearly, we have a problem. But Oliver Wendell Holmes recognized that fact many years ago:

"I firmly believe that if the entire *materia medica* as now used could be sunk to the bottom of the sea, it would be all the better for mankind — and all the worse for the fishes."

Index

About Doctor William Campbell Douglass II

Dr. Douglass reveals medical truths, and deceptions, often at risk of being labeled heretical. He is consumed by a passion for living a long healthy life, and wants his readers to share that passion. Their health and well-being comes first. He is anti-dogmatic, and unwavering in his dedication to improve the quality of life of his readers. He has been called "the conscience of modern medicine," a "medical maverick," and has been voted "Doctor of the Year" by the National Health Federation. His medical experiences are far reaching-from battling malaria in Central America - to fighting deadly epidemics at his own health clinic in Africa - to flying with U.S. Navy crews as a flight surgeon - to working for 10 years in emergency medicine here in the States. These learning experiences, not to mention his keen storytelling ability and wit, make Dr. Douglass' newsletters (Daily Dose and Real Health) and books uniquely interesting and fun to read. He shares his no-frills, no-bull approach to health care, often amazing his readers by telling them to ignore many widely-hyped good-health practices (like staying away from red meat, avoiding coffee, and eating like a bird), and start living again by eating REAL food, taking some inexpensive supplements, and doing the pleasurable things that make life livable. Readers get all this, plus they learn how to burn fat, prevent cancer, boost libido, and so much more. And, Dr. Douglass is not afraid to challenge the latest studies that come out, and share the real story with his readers. Dr. William C. Douglass has led a colorful, rebellious, and crusading life. Not many physicians would dare put their professional reputations on the line as many times as this courageous healer has. A vocal opponent of "business-as-usual" medicine, Dr. Douglass has championed patients' rights and physician commitment to wellness throughout his career. This dedicated physician has repeatedly gone far beyond the call of duty in his work to spread the truth about alternative therapies. For a full year, he endured economic and physical hardship to work with physicians at the Pasteur Institute in St. Petersburg, Russia, where advanced research on photoluminescence was being conducted. Dr. Douglass comes from a distinguished family of physicians. He is the fourth generation Douglass to practice medicine, and his son is also a physician. Dr. Douglass graduated from the University of Rochester, the Miami School of Medicine, and the Naval School of Aviation and Space Medicine.

You want to protect those you love from the health dangers the authorities aren't telling you about, and learn the incredible cures that they've scorned and ignored?

Subscribe to the free Daily Dose updates "...the straight scoop about health, medicine, and politics." by sending an e-mail to real_sub@agoramail.net with the word "subscribe" in the subject line.

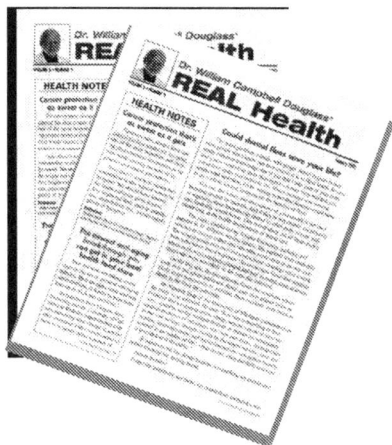

If you knew of a procedure that could save thousands, maybe millions, of people dying from AIDS, cancer, and other dreaded killers....

Would you cover it up?

It's unthinkable that what could be the best solution ever to stopping the world's killer diseases is being ignored, scorned, and rejected. But that is exactly what's happening right now.

The procedure is called "photoluminescence". It's a thoroughly tested, proven therapy that uses the healing power of the light to perform almost miraculous cures.

This remarkable treatment works its incredible cures by stimulating the body's own immune responses. That's why it cures so many ailments--and why it's been especially effective against AIDS! Yet, 50 years ago, it virtually disappeared from the halls of medicine.

Why has this incredible cure been ignored by the medical authorities of this country? You'll find the shocking answer here in the pages of this new edition of Into the Light. Now available with the blood irradiation Instrument Diagram and a complete set of instructions for building your own "Treatment Device". Also includes details on how to use this unique medical instrument.

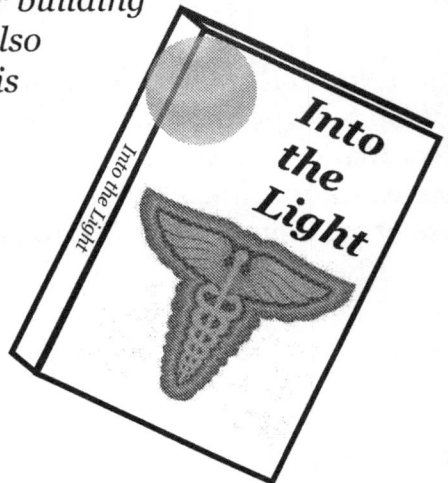

Into the Light

Into
the
Light

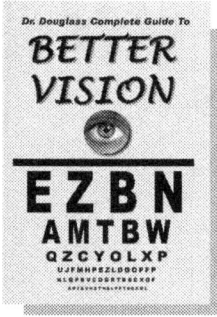

Dr. Douglass' Complete Guide to Better Vision

A report about eyesight and what can be done to improve it naturally. But I've also included information about how the eye works, brief descriptions of various common eye conditions, traditional remedies to eye problems, and a few simple suggestions that may help you maintain your eyesight for years to come.
-William Campbell Douglass II, MD

The Hypertension Report.
Say Good Bye to High Blood Pressure.

An estimated 50 million Americans have high blood pressure. Often called the "silent killer" because it may not cause symptoms until the patient has suffered serious damage to the arterial system. Diet, exercise, potassium supplements chelation therapy and practically anything but drugs is the way to go and alternatives are discussed in this report.

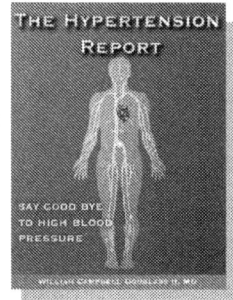

Grandma Bell's A To Z Guide To Healing With Herbs.

This book is all about - coming home. What I once believed to be old wives' tales - stories long destroyed by the new world of science - actually proved to be the best treatment for many of the common ailments you and I suffer through. So I put a few of them together in this book with the sincere hope that Grandma Bell's wisdom will help you recover your common sense, and take responsibility for your own health. -William Campbell Douglass II, MD

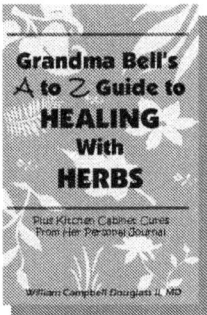

Prostate Problems:
Safe, Simple, Effective Relief for Men over 50.

Don't be frightened into surgery or drugs you may not need. First, get the facts about prostate problems... know all your options, so you can make the best decisions. This fully documented report explains the dangers of conventional treatments, and gives you alternatives that could save you more than just money!

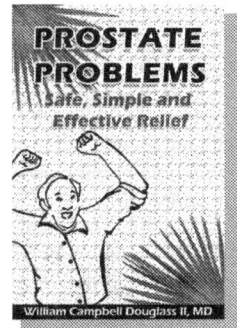

Color me Healthy
The Healing Powers
of Colors

"He's crazy!"
"He's got to be a quack!"
"Who gave this guy his medical license?"
"He's a nut case!"

In case you're wondering, those are the reactions you'll probably get if you show your doctor this report. I know the idea of healing many common ailments simply by exposing them to colored light sounds far-fetched, but when you see the evidence, you'll agree that color is truly an amazing medical breakthrough.

When I first heard the stories,
I reacted much the same way.
But the evidence so
convinced me, that I had to
try color therapy in my practice.
My results were truly amazing.

-William Campbell Douglass II, MD

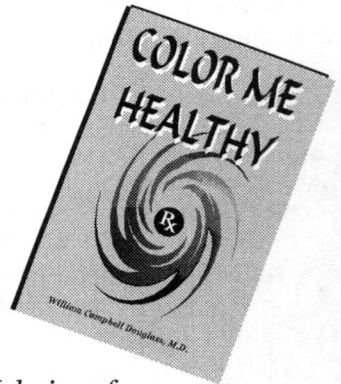

Order your complete set of Roscolene filters (choice of 3 sizes) to be used with the "Color Me Healthy" therapy. The eleven Roscolene filters are # 809, 810, 818, 826, 828, 832, 859, 861, 866, 871, and 877. The filters come with protective separator sheets between each filter. The color names and the Roscolene filter(s) used to produce that particular color, are printed on a card included with the filters and a set of instructions on how to fit them to a lamp.

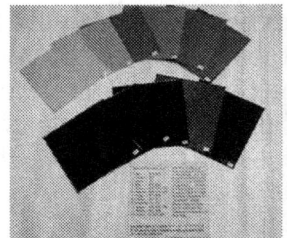

What Is Going on Here?

Peroxides are supposed to be bad for you. Free radicals and all that. But now we hear that hydrogen peroxide is good for us. Hydrogen peroxide will put extra oxygen in your blood. There's no doubt about that. Hydrogen peroxide costs pennies. So if you can get oxygen into the blood cheaply and safely, maybe cancer (which doesn't like oxygen), emphysema, AIDS, and many other terrible diseases can be treated effectively. Intravenous hydrogen peroxide rapidly relieves allergic reactions, influenza symptoms, and acute viral infections.

No one expects to live forever. But we would all like to have a George Burns finish. The prospect of finishing life in a nursing home after abandoning your tricycle in the mobile home park is not appealing. Then comes the loss of control of vital functions the ultimate humiliation. Is life supposed to be from tricycle to tricycle and diaper to diaper? You come into this world crying, but do you have to leave crying? I don't believe you do. And you won't either after you see the evidence. Sounds too good to be true, doesn't it? Read on and decide for yourself.

-William Campbell Douglass II, MD

Rhino Publishing S.A.
www.rhinopublish.com

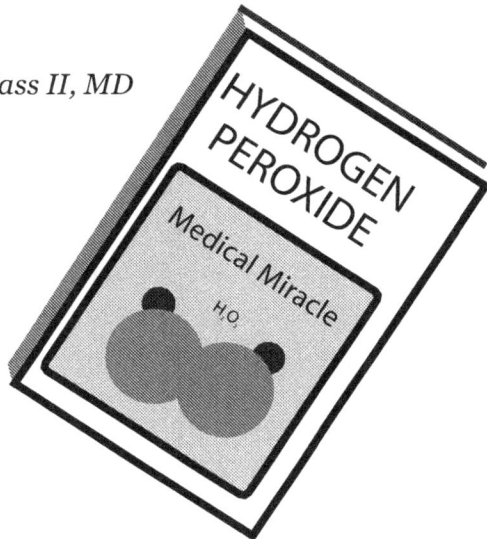

HYDROGEN PEROXIDE
Medical Miracle
H_2O

Don't drink your milk!

If you knew what we know about milk... BLEECHT! All that pasteurization, homogenization and processing is not only cooking all the nutrients right out of your favorite drink. It's also adding toxic levels of vitamin D.

This fascinating book tells the whole story about milk. How it once was nature's perfect food...how "raw," unprocessed milk can heal and boost your immune system ... why you can't buy it legally in this country anymore, and what we could do to change that.

Dr. "Douglass traveled all over the world, tasting all kinds of milk from all kinds of cows, poring over dusty research books in ancient libraries far from home, to write this light-hearted but scientifically sound book.

Rhino Publishing, S.A.
www.rhinopublish.com

The Milk Book

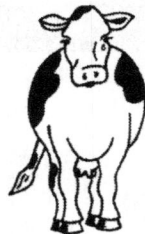

William Campbell Douglass II, MD

Eat Your Cholesterol!

Eat Meat, Drink Milk, Spread The Butter- And Live Longer!
How to Live off the Fat of the Land and Feel Great.

Americans are being saturated with anti-cholesterol propaganda. If you watch very much television, you're probably one of the millions of Americans who now has a terminal case of cholesterol phobia. The propaganda is relentless and is often designed to produce fear and loathing of this worst of all food contaminants. You never hear the food propagandists bragging about their product being fluoride-free or aluminum-free, two of our truly serious food-additive problems. But cholesterol, an essential nutrient, not proven to be harmful in any quantity, is constantly pilloried as a menace to your health. If you don't use corn oil, Fleischmann's margarine, and Egg Beaters, you're going straight to atherosclerosis hell with stroke, heart attack, and premature aging -- and so are your kids. Never feel guilty about what you eat again! Dr. Douglass shows you why red meat, eggs, and dairy products aren't the dietary demons we're told they are. But beware: This scientifically sound report goes against all the "common wisdom" about the foods you should eat. Read with an open mind.

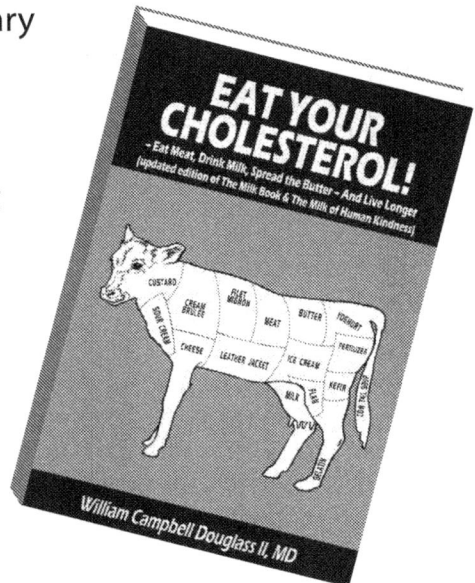

Rhino Publishing, S.A.
www.rhinopublish.com

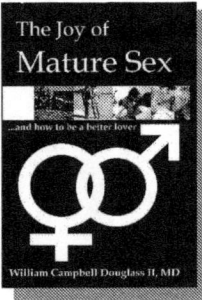

The Joy of Mature Sex and How to Be a Better Lover

Humans are very confused about what makes good sex. But I believe humans have more to offer each other than this total licentiousness common among animals. We're talking about mature sex. The kind of sex that made this country great.

Stop Aging or Slow the Process How Exercise With Oxygen Therapy (EWOT) Can Help

EWOT (pronounced ee-watt) stands for Exercise With Oxygen Therapy. This method of prolonging your life is so simple and you can do it at home at a minimal cost. When your cells don't get enough oxygen, they degenerate and die and so you degenerate and die. It's as simple as that.

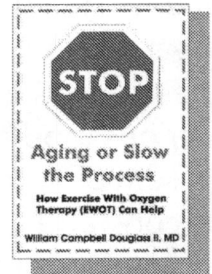

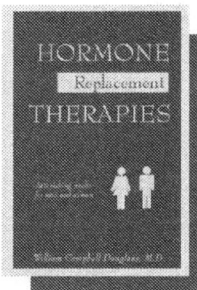

Hormone Replacement Therapies: Astonishing Results For Men And Women

It is accurate to say that when the endocrine glands start to fail, you start to die. We are facing a sea change in longevity and health in the elderly. Now, with the proper supplemental hormones, we can slow the aging process and, in many cases, reverse some of the signs and symptoms of aging.

Add 10 Years to Your Life With some "best of" Dr. Douglass' writings.

To add ten years to your life, you need to have the right attitude about health and an understanding of the health industry and what it's feeding you. Following the established line on many health issues could make you very sick or worse! Achieve dynamic health with this collection of some of the "best of" Dr. Douglass' newsletters.

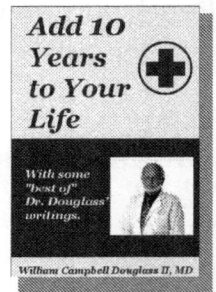

How did AIDS become one of the Greatest Biological Disasters in the History of Mankind?

GET THE FACTS

AIDS and BIOLOGICAL WARFARE covers the history of plagues from the past to today's global confrontation with AIDS, the Prince of Plagues. Completely documented *AIDS and BIOLOGICAL WARFARE* helps you make your own decisions about how to survive in a world ravaged by this horrible plague.

You will learn that AIDS is not a naturally occuring disease process as you have been led to believe, but a man-made biological nightmare that has been unleashed and is now threatening the very existence of human life on the planet.

There is a smokescreen of misinformation clouding the AIDS issue. Now, for the first time, learn the truth about the nature of the crisis our planet faces: its origin -- how AIDS is really transmited and alternatives for treatment. Find out what they are not telling you about AIDS and Biological Warfare, and how to protect yourself and your loved ones. AIDS is a serious problem worldwide, but it is no longer the major threat. You need to know the whole story. To protect yourself, you must know the truth about biological warfare.

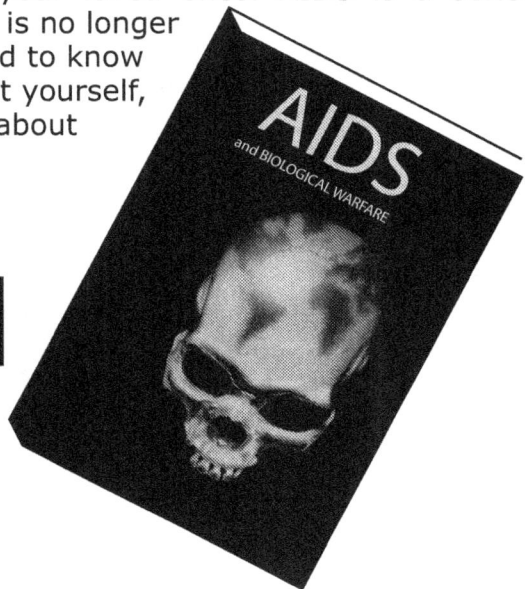

PAINFUL DILEMMA

Are we fighting the wrong war?

We are spending millions on the war against drugs while we
should be fighting the war against pain with those drugs!

As you will read in this book, the war on drugs was lost a long time ago and,
when it comes to the war against pain, pain is winning! An article in USA Today
(11/20/02) reveals that dying patients are not getting relief from pain. It seems
the doctors are torn between fear of the government, certainly justified, and a
clinging to old and out dated ideas about pain, which is NOT justified.

A group called Last Acts, a coalition of health-care groups, has released a very
discouraging study of all 50 states that nearly half of the 1.6 million Americans
living in nursing homes suffer from untreated pain. They said that life was being
extended but it amounted to little more than "extended pain and suffering."

This book offers insight into the history of pain treatment and the current failed
philosophies of contemporary medicine. Plus it describes some of today's most
advanced treatments for alleviating certain kinds of pain. This book is not another
"self-help" book touting home remedies; rather, Painful Dilemma: Patients in
Pain -- People in Prison, takes a hard look at where we've gone wrong and what
we (you) can do to help a loved one who is living with chronic pain.

The second half of this book is a must read if you value your freedom. We now
have the ridiculous and tragic situation of people
in pain living in a government-created hell by
restriction of narcotics and people in prison for
trying to bring pain relief by the selling of
narcotics to the suffering. The end result of the
"war on drugs" has been to create the greatest
and most destructive cartel in history, so great,
in fact, that the drug Mafia now controls most
of the world economy.

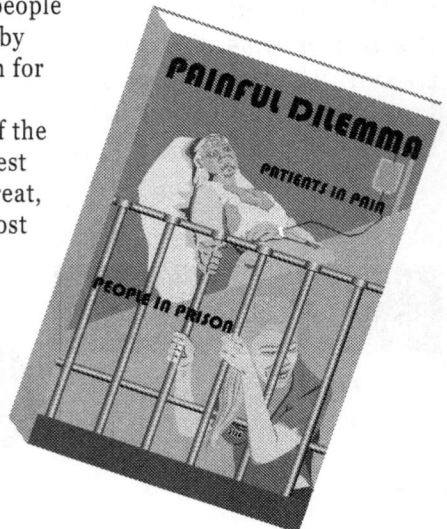

Rhino Publishing S.A.
www.rhinopublish.com

Live the Adventure!

Why would anyone in their right mind put everything they own in storage and move to Russia, of all places?! But when maverick physician Bill Douglass left a profitable medical practice in a peaceful mountaintop town to pursue "pure medical truth".... none of us who know him well was really surprised.

After All, anyone who's braved the outermost reaches of darkest Africa, the mean streets of Johannesburg and New York, and even a trip to Washington to testify before the Senate, wouldn't bat and eye at ducking behind the Iron Curtain for a little medical reconnaissance!

Enjoy this imaginative, funny, dedicated man's tales of wonder and woe as he treks through a year in St. Petersburg, working on a cure for the world's killer diseases. We promise --

YOU WON'T BE BORED!

Rhino Publishing S.A.
www.rhinopublish.com

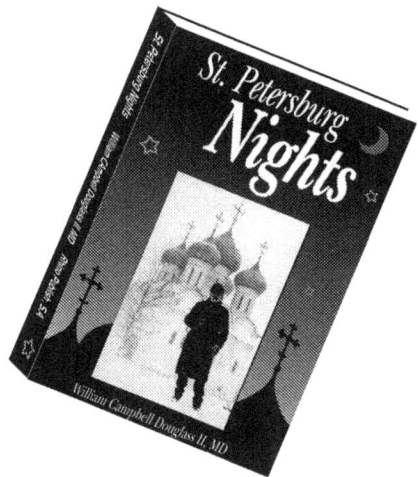

St. Petersburg Nights

William Campbell Douglass II, MD

THE SMOKER'S PARADOX
THE HEALTH BENEFITS OF TOBACCO!

The benefits of smoking tobacco have been common knowledge for centuries. From sharpening mental acuity to maintaining optimal weight, the relatively small risks of smoking have always been outweighed by the substantial improvement to mental and physical health. Hysterical attacks on tobacco notwithstanding, smokers always weigh the good against the bad and puff away or quit according to their personal preferences. Now the same anti-tobacco enterprise that has spent billions demonizing the pleasure of smoking is providing additional reasons to smoke. Alzheimer's, Parkinson's, Tourette's Syndrome, even schizophrenia and cocaine addiction are disorders that are alleviated by tobacco. Add in the still inconclusive indication that tobacco helps to prevent colon and prostate cancer and the endorsement for smoking tobacco by the medical establishment is good news for smokers and non-smokers alike. Of course the revelation that tobacco is good for you is ruined by the pharmaceutical industry's plan to substitute the natural and relatively inexpensive tobacco plant with their overpriced and ineffective nicotine substitutions. Still, when all is said and done, the positive revelations regarding tobacco are very good reasons indeed to keep lighting those cigars - but only 4 a day!

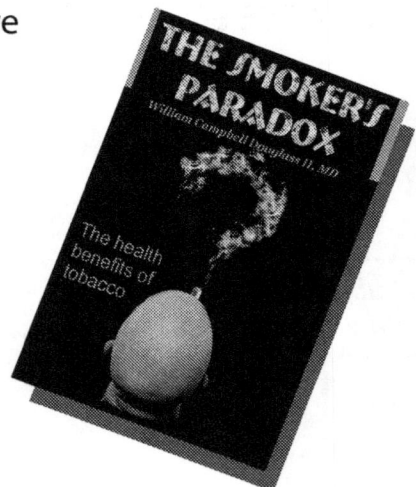

Rhino Publishing, S.A
www.rhinopublish.com

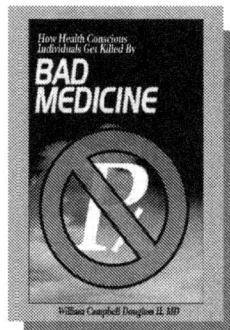

Bad Medicine
How Individuals Get Killed By Bad Medicine.

Do you really need that new prescription or that overnight stay in the hospital? In this report, Dr. Douglass reveals the common medical practices and misconceptions endangering your health. Best of all, he tells you the pointed (but very revealing!) questions your doctor prays you never ask. Interesting medical facts about popular remedies are revealed.

Dangerous Legal Drugs
The Poisons in Your Medicine Chest.

If you knew what we know about the most popular prescription and over-the-counter drugs, you'd be sick. That's why Dr. Douglass wrote this shocking report about the poisons in your medicine chest. He gives you the low-down on different categories of drugs. Everything from painkillers and cold remedies to tranquilizers and powerful cancer drugs.

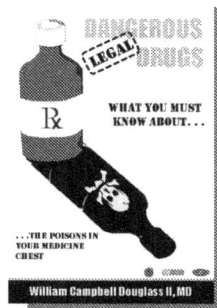

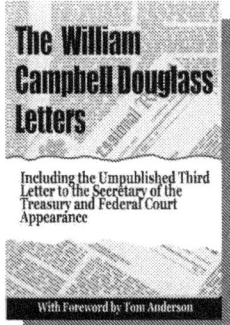

The William Campbell Douglass Letters.
Expose of Government Machinations
(Vietnam War).

THE WILLIAM CAMPBELL DOUGLASS LETTERS. Dr. Douglass' Defense in 1968 Tax Case and Expose of Government Machinations during the Vietnam War.

The Eagle's Feather. A Novel of
International Political Intrigue.

Although The Eagle's Feather is a work of fiction set in the 1970's, it is built, as with most fiction, on a framework of plausibility and background information. This is a fiction book that could not have been written were it not for various ominous aspects, which pose a clear and present danger to the security of the United States.

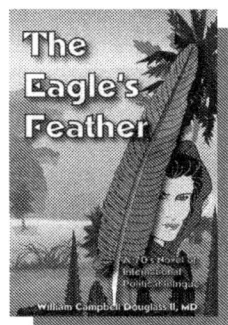

Rhino Publishing

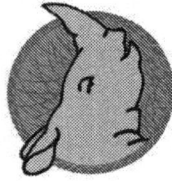

ORDER FORM

PURCHASER INFORMATION

Purchaser's Name (Please Print): _____

Shipping Address (Do not use a P.O. Box): _____

City: _____ State/Prov.: _____ Country: _____

Zip/Postal Code: _____ Telephone No.: _____ Fax No.: _____

E-Mail Address (if interested in receiving free e-Books when available): _____

CREDIT CARD INFO (CIRCLE ONE):

MASTERCARD, VISA, AMERICAN EXPRESS, DISCOVER, JCB, DINER'S CLUB, CARTE BLANCHE.

Charge my Card -> Number #: _____ Exp.: _____

*Security Code: _____ * Required for all MasterCard, Visa and American Express purchases. For your security, we require that you enter your card's verification number. The verification number is also called a CCV number. This code is the 3 digits farthest right in the signature field on the back of your VISA/MC, or the 4 digits to the right on the front of your American Express card. Your credit card statement will show **a different name than Rhino Publishing** as the vendor.

WE DO NOT share your private information, we use 3ʳᵈ party credit card processing service to process your order only.

ADDITIONAL INFORMATION

If your shipping address is not the same as your credit card billing address, please indicate your card billing address here.

Name on the card _____ Type of card: _____

Billing Address: _____

City: _____ State/Prov.: _____ Zip/Postal Code: _____

Fax a copy of this order to:
RHINO PUBLISHING, S.A.
1-888-317-6767 or International #: + 416-352-5126

To order by mail, send your payment by first class mail only to the following address. Please include a copy of this order form. Make your check or bank drafts (NO postal money order) payable to RHINO PUBLISHING, S.A. and mail to:

Rhino Publishing, S.A.
Attention: PTY 5048
P.O. Box 025724
Miami, FL.
USA 33102

Digital E-books also available online: www.rhinopublish.com

Rhino Publishing

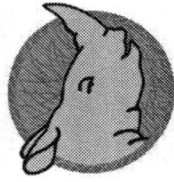

ORDER FORM

Purchaser's Name (Please Print): _____

I would like to order the following paperback book of Dr. Douglass (Alternative Medicine Books):

___	X	9962-636-04-3	Add 10 Years to Your Life. With some "best of" Dr. Douglass writings.	$13.99 $_____
___	X	9962-636-07-8	AIDS and Biological Warfare. What They Are Not Telling You!	$17.99 $_____
___	X	9962-636-09-4	Bad Medicine. How Individuals Get Killed By Bad Medicine.	$11.99 $_____
___	X	9962-636-10-8	Color Me Healthy. The Healing Power of Colors.	$11.99 $_____
___	X	9962-636 -XX-X	Color Filters for Color Me Healthy. 11 Basic Roscolene Filters for Lamps.	$21.89 $_____
___	X	9962-636-15-9	Dangerous Legal Drugs. The Poisons in Your Medicine Chest.	$13.99 $_____
___	X	9962-636-18-3	Dr. Douglass' Complete Guide to Better Vision. Improve eyesight naturally.	$11.99 $_____
___	X	9962-636-19-1	Eat Your Cholesterol! How to Live off the Fat of the Land and Feel Great.	$11.99 $_____
___	X	9962-636-12-4	Grandma Bell's A To Z Guide To Healing. Her Kitchen Cabinet Cures.	$14.99 $_____
___	X	9962-636-22-1	Hormone Replacement Therapies. Astonishing Results For Men & Women	$11.99 $_____
___	X	9962-636-25-6	Hydrogen Peroxide: One of the Most Underused Medical Miracle.	$15.99 $_____
___	X	9962-636-27-2	Into the Light. New Edition with Blood Irradiation Instrument Instructions.	$19.99 $_____
___	X	9962-636-54-X	Milk Book. The Classic on the Nutrition of Milk and How to Benefit from it.	$17.99 $_____

_____	X	9962-636-00-0	Painful Dilemma - Patients in Pain - People in Prison.	$17.99	$ _____
_____	X	9962-636-32-9	Prostate Problems. Safe, Simple, Effective Relief for Men over 50.	$11.99	$ _____
_____	X	9962-636-34-5	St. Petersburg Nights. Enlightening Story of Life and Science in Russia.	$17.99	$ _____
_____	X	9962-636-37-X	Stop Aging or Slow the Process. Exercise With Oxygen Therapy Can Help.	$11.99	$ _____
_____	X	9962-636-60-4	The Hypertension Report. Say Good Bye to High Blood Pressure.	$11.99	$ _____
_____	X	9962-636-48-5	The Joy of Mature Sex and How to Be a Better Lover...	$13.99	$ _____
_____	X	9962-636-43-4	The Smoker's Paradox: Health Benefits of Tobacco.	$14.99	$ _____

Political Books:

_____	X	9962-636-40-X	The Eagle's Feather. A 70's Novel of International Political Intrigue.	$15.99	$ _____
_____	X	9962-636-46-9	The W. C. D. Letters. Expose of Government Machinations (Vietnam War).	$11.99	$ _____

SUB-TOTAL: $ _____

ADD $5.00 HANDLING FOR YOUR ORDER: $ 5.00 $ 5.00

_____ X ADD $2.50 SHIPPING FOR EACH ITEM ON ORDER: $ 2.50 $ _____

NOTE THAT THE MINIMUM SHIPPING AND HANDLING IS $7.50 FOR 1 BOOK ($5.00 + $2.50)
For order shipped outside the US, add $5.00 per item

_____ X ADD $5.00 S. & H. OR EACH ITEM ON ORDER (INTERNATIONAL ORDERS ONLY) $ 5.00 $ _____
Allow up to 21 days for delivery (we will call you about back orders if any)

TOTAL: $ _____

Fax a copy of this order to: 1-888-317-6767 or Int'l + 416-352-5126
or mail to: Rhino Publishing, S.A. Attention: PTY 5048 P.O. Box 025724, Miami, FL., 33102 USA
Digital E-books also available online: www.rhinopublish.com

www.ingramcontent.com/pod-product-compliance
Lightning Source LLC
Chambersburg PA
CBHW032101020426
42335CB00011B/440